The
LONGEVITY
DIET

The
LONGEVITY
DIET

Discover the New Science to
Slow Ageing, Fight Disease,
and Manage Your Weight

Valter Longo, PhD

MICHAEL JOSEPH
an imprint of
PENGUIN BOOKS

MICHAEL JOSEPH

UK | USA | Canada | Ireland | Australia
India | New Zealand | South Africa

Michael Joseph is part of the Penguin Random House group of companies
whose addresses can be found at global.penguinrandomhouse.com

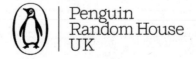

First published in Italy 2016 by Antonio Vallardi Editore
Published in the United States of America by Avery 2018
Published in Great Britain by Michael Joseph 2018
001

Photo on page 104 of baby boy used with permission of irin-k/Shutterstock.com. Photo on page 104
of happy couple used with the permission of T-Design/Shutterstock.com. Illustrations on page 143 used
with the permission of Ilinova Tetiana/Shutterstock.com and Voinau Pavel/Shutterstock.com."Fasting
Transformed Me After Medicine Failed" by Jenni Russell on page 206–207 © *The Times* / News
Syndication. Image on page 30 from "Evolutionary Medicine: From Dwarf Model Systems to Healthy
Centenarians?" by Valter D. Longo, Caleb E. Finch, in *Science*, February 28, 2003: vol 299, issue 5611,
p. 1342. Reprinted with permission. Mouse photo © Dr. Michael Bonkowski AAAS.

Printed in Great Britain by Clays Ltd, St Ives plc

A CIP catalogue record for this book is available from the British Library

ISBN: 978–1–405–93394–0

www.greenpenguin.co.uk

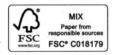

MIX
Paper from
responsible sources
FSC® C018179

Penguin Random House is committed to a
sustainable future for our business, our readers
and our planet. This book is made from Forest
Stewardship Council® certified paper.

To my mother, Angelina; my father, Carmelo;
my brother, Claudio; and my sister, Patrizia.

And to those seeking solutions, knowledge, and hope.

Contents

Introduction xi

Chapter 1

Caruso's Fountain 1

Chapter 2

Aging, Programmed Longevity, and Juventology 16

Chapter 3

The Five Pillars 37

Chapter 4

The Longevity Diet 49

Chapter 5

Exercise and Healthy Longevity 87

Chapter 6

Fasting-Mimicking Diets, Weight Management, and Healthy Longevity 96

Chapter 7

**Nutrition and Fasting-Mimicking Diets in
Cancer Prevention and Treatment** 117

Chapter 8

**Nutrition, FMD, and Diabetes Prevention
and Treatment** 138

Chapter 9

**FMD, Nutrition, and Cardiovascular Disease
Prevention and Treatment** 160

Chapter 10

**FMD and Nutrition in the Prevention and
Treatment of Alzheimer's and other
Neurodegenerative Diseases** 176

Chapter 11

**FMD and Nutrition in the Prevention and
Treatment of Inflammatory and
Autoimmune Diseases** 194

Chapter 12

How to Stay Young 211

Appendix A: Longevity Diet Two-Week Meal Plan 219
Appendix B: Food Sources of Vitamins and Minerals 253
Acknowledgments 269
Notes 273
Index 287

The
LONGEVITY
DIET

Introduction

LONGEVITY, THE FOUNTAIN OF LIFE, the secrets to eternal youth—they have fascinated us from our earliest civilizations. And they have deeply fascinated me since I was a teenager. Back then I wanted to become a rock star, and I was sure I would always be a professional musician, but my passion to discover the secrets of longevity and how they could revolutionize medicine wouldn't be drowned out, no matter how fantastic a rock career appeared to be. When I was a sophomore in college, I decided to put music to the side and dedicate myself to science so that I could study the processes by which we age. Three decades later, I still play guitar, but I spend the majority of my time working as the director of the University of Southern California (USC) Longevity Institute in Los Angeles and the Program on Longevity and Cancer at IFOM (Molecular Oncology FIRC Institute) in Milan, where I combine studies of centenarians with epidemiological studies of populations, clinical trials, and basic research to understand how to help people live long lives.

But it's not just the idea of living longer that has driven me; it's living *healthy* longer, staying vibrant and youthful beyond the traditional life expectancy. To achieve this, my laboratories performed decades of cellular, animal, and human studies focused on maximizing function (learning, memory, physical fitness, etc.) and on the prevention and treatment of diseases, with a special focus on cancer, diabetes, and cardiovascular disease as well as autoimmune and neurodegenerative disorders. Contrary to the notion that if we live longer we will extend the "sickness" period, our data indicate that by understanding how the human body is maintained while young, we can stay fully functional into our nineties, hundreds, and beyond. One of the primary ways to achieve this is to exploit our body's innate ability to regenerate itself at the cellular and organ levels. Unfortunately, the modern diet, and the constant consumption that characterizes the way so much of the first world eats, keeps these built-in mechanisms permanently switched off, leaving us prematurely vulnerable to disease and degeneration beginning in our thirties and forties. But as I've discovered over the past thirty years of research, that switch can be turned back on rather easily. The difficult part has been figuring out a way to do it that is feasible and safe for everyone.

Let me back up. I was sixteen when I first came to America from Genoa (hometown of Christopher Columbus), in the northwest of Italy. That's where I was born and raised, though I spent my summers in Calabria, the southern Italian region where my parents came from. Harboring my dreams of fame and fortune as a rock star—and having driven neighbors in my building crazy for long enough with loud electric guitars—I arrived in Chicago to live with an aunt and pursue my music studies. Along with the thriving music scene, and some of the best blues in the nation, I was exposed for the first time to the American diet. Having grown up in two regions with some of the healthiest cuisines in the world and never really having thought about it, I was amazed at the giant portions, the huge amounts of meat and cheese consumed at almost every meal, the sugary drinks and snacks so readily available. The other thing I noticed was that my Italian relatives living in Chicago were developing diabetes, heart disease, and other ailments uncommon to the family back home. At the time, I didn't think much of it, but later these exposures motivated me and helped me solidify hypotheses about diet, diseases, and longevity.

By the time I got to the University of North Texas just outside of Dallas a few years later to continue my music education, my fascination with aging had taken hold. All my friends who were approaching or past thirty were starting to lament getting old. But something else, maybe my having been in the room when my grandfather died, was stuck in my head, waiting for an opportunity to guide me in a new direction. As much as I loved music, in my second year as an undergraduate I realized that what I really wanted to do with my life was study how people stay young, so I moved to the biochemistry department to begin studying aging. Four years later, I entered one of the best programs for the biology of aging, the pathology PhD programs at the University of California, Los Angeles, and the laboratory of Roy Walford, MD, who at the time was the world's leading expert on nutrition and longevity, a field that was just beginning to come into its own. The rest is history.

I have now been researching healthy longevity for more than thirty years, studying the links between nutrition and the genes that regulate cellular protection and regeneration. *The Longevity Diet* collects what I have learned and puts it into a simple program anyone can live by. It is as simple as adopting the daily nutritional regimen I outline and combining it periodically (two to twelve times per year, depending on your general health) with my fasting-mimicking diet (FMD), which is exactly what it sounds like: a diet that mimics a fast, providing the benefits of fasting without the deprivation and hunger. Combining these two elements, I have discovered, can protect, regenerate, and rejuvenate the body to keep us young and healthy longer. This is achieved in part by turning back the biological aging clock, which means that these diets can be adopted by relatively young people to help delay aging and prevent disease, and also by older individuals to help them return to a more youthful state. The FMD is also clinically proven to stimulate the loss of abdominal fat while conserving muscle and bone mass. These benefits are generated by switching on the human body's own remarkable ability to activate stem cells and regenerate parts of cells, systems, and organs, leading to a reduction of risk factors for many diseases. In the chapters that follow, I will explain first *why* it works, then *how* it works. I will also explain how we took advantage of scientific and clinical experience to make nutritional strategies safe and feasible while minimizing the need for drastic dietary changes. Our dietary interventions are now recommended by thousands of doctors in the United States, Europe, and Asia.

Among other things that I believe set this book apart from the thousands of other diet and wellness books out there is that it is based on a solid multidisciplinary foundation. We are constantly bombarded with new science that demonizes or exalts one food or another. For this reason, I devised a methodology that would ensure the widest possible scientific basis for my recommendations. I call this method the Five Pillars of Longevity. These pillars do not refer to specific interventions such as diet and exercise, but to five disciplines that provide the foundation for my nutrition program: 1) basic/juventology research (juventology, as I will explain, is the science of staying young); 2) epidemiology; 3) clinical studies; 4) studies of centenarians; and 5) the understanding of complex systems (like cars, for example). By thus providing the widest, most solid grounds possible for dietary and exercise recommendations, we not only ensure their efficacy, but we also reduce to a minimum the chance that a future set of studies will drastically alter them. The past thirty years of research, and learning from many scientists in these different fields, have allowed me to build a system that I believe is solid enough that you can use it for life.

My search for the secrets to youthful longevity has led me all around the world, from Los Angeles to the Andes of southern Ecuador; from Okinawa, Japan, to Russia; from the Netherlands to southern Germany. But ultimately it led me back to Italy. Though I had no idea of this when I was growing up, the part of northern Italy where I was born and raised happens to be home to one of the highest percentages of people over age sixty-five in the world (28.3 percent, according to the Italian National Institute of Statistics in 2016), and the region in the south where I spent every summer of my childhood has, we discovered, one of the highest proportions of centenarians worldwide. It has been a very surprising coincidence but also a confirmation and privilege of my life's work to take my studies back to where I grew up and be able to see that part of the world again through the eyes of people who have lived long, healthy, and full lives there. Inspired by all my long-lived friends back home and around the world, this book is for anyone who wishes to join their ranks.

A Note on Proceeds and Products

This book gives you the advantage of many years of research into how to live long and healthy lives, but there is another benefit; with 100 percent of my book royalties going to charity, you'll also be helping to fund valuable research through organizations like the Create Cures Foundation (www.createcures.org), a nonprofit organization I founded to support people with advanced-stage or complex diseases in need of integrative and more effective treatments. Every day I get emails from people who have been diagnosed with serious diseases—cancer, autoimmune and metabolic disorders, neurodegenerative diseases, etc.—seeking options beyond the standard treatments offered by their doctors. Unfortunately, professional guidelines, fear of legal action, heavy case-loads, and the complexity of illness work to keep doctors narrowly focused on standard-of-care treatments, and often patients aren't given integrative options even if they ask. As I spent time with clinicians working on innovative therapies for cancer and other diseases, it became clear that they needed researchers like me to help them offer integrative interventions that could be safe, built on solid research, and advantageous to their patients, who in many cases do not have the option of waiting years for the end of large clinical trials.

This is how I came to start the Create Cures Foundation. Our mission is to make evidence-based information available to the public, to empower those who want to complement traditional treatments with reliable, scientifically based and clinically tested strategies to improve the efficacy of the therapy but also reduce its side effects. Our goal is not to diminish the role of medical doctors in patient care, but to enhance it by providing information on integrative approaches supported by strong animal and clinical data. We live in a time when funding for research is getting tighter, with very little going to creative or alternative ideas, which is why my profits from the sale of this book will go straight to the Create Cures Foundation and other nonprofit universities and institutes. So go ahead and buy more copies! Give them to your friends and family. You'll be helping whomever you give it to, and you'll also be directly funding our ongoing research into aging, cancer, Alzheimer's, Parkinson's, cardiovascular disease, multiple sclerosis, Crohn's disease and colitis, and type 1 and type 2 diabetes. (I list these particular diseases because we have performed basic research on all of them, and are planning or have started, and in some cases completed, clinical trials with documented success.) We are committed to transforming research into improved, applicable therapies as rapidly as we can by thinking broadly and creatively. Our approach is to work with as many leading hospitals and research institutes as possible—at the moment these include Harvard, the Mayo Clinic, Charité–University Medicine Berlin, Leiden University, and University of Genova, among many others—even as we continue to perform our own basic research and clinical trials at USC's Leonard Davis School of Gerontology and Keck Medical Center, one of the largest and best university hospitals in the United States, and at the IFOM Cancer Research Institute, in Milan, Italy. You can receive updates on our research, including upcoming clinical trials, on my Facebook page, @profvalterlongo, and at www.createcures.org.

Virtually every one of the patients who wrote to me asked the same question: having heard that my fasting-mimicking diet can bring all the benefits of fasting without the actual fasting part, they want to know what they can eat while on the "fast." In response, and in order to make the FMD available as well as safe and effective for everyone, I started a company called L-Nutra (www.l-nutra.com). With support from the US National Cancer Institute, the National Institute on Aging, and other funding agencies, we first developed a clinically tested FMD for cancer patients (Chemolieve®), then one for everyone (ProLon®). One hundred percent of my shares in L-Nutra are committed to the Create Cures Foundation and other nonprofit organizations involved in research relevant to our mission. (I receive neither a salary nor a consulting fee from L-Nutra—though in the interest of full disclosure, I do receive minimal expense reimbursement.) Although I do not directly make pricing decisions, I am committed to ensuring that L-Nutra's products are as affordable as possible without compromising quality or the company's ability to grow and make its products available around the world.

ProLon is already available through the L-Nutra website in the

United States and is recommended by a network of physicians and other healthcare professionals. Chemolieve is currently being tested at several leading cancer centers, including USC, the Mayo Clinic, and Leiden University, and there is a long list of institutions waiting to test different FMDs for many diseases and conditions as soon as funding becomes available.

Many eager patients have asked whether it's necessary to buy the products and use them under supervision, or whether they can just do the FMD themselves at home. I always answer the question by first reminding people that half of my program, the everyday Longevity Diet part, consists of foods that can be purchased in any supermarket and does not require supervision or specially formulated products. The Longevity Diet alone will help prevent and treat many diseases, and will also reduce the recommended frequency of the FMD. That said, when it comes to the FMD, after years of experience with patients doing it in different ways—with the product and without; under supervision and not—I've concluded that it *should* really be done with the clinically tested product and preferably under the supervision of a registered dietitian or physician. Although all ingredients are completely safe, fasting and FMDs have powerful effects that can be turned against aging and diseases but that can also result in side effects, in some cases severe. The use of the clinically tested product, along with the right screening and supervision, will guarantee maximum safety and efficacy. (The great majority of experts recommend that prolonged fasting periods—anything more than one day—be done only in clinics under the supervision of specialized medical personnel.) The clinically tested ProLon FMD will allow most people to do the diet at home. If you are healthy and have the means and access to consult a registered dietitian before undertaking the FMD, especially for the first time, it is strongly recommended that you do so. If you have been diagnosed with a disease, you must have the approval of your doctor. You can find information and specialists on L-Nutra's website.

Chapter 1

Caruso's Fountain

Back to Molochio

Drive an hour and a half north from the southernmost tip of Italy and you'll reach a little town called Molochio in the region of Calabria. Its name is probably derived from the Greek word *molokhē*, meaning "mallow," which is a medicinal plant with a bright purple flower. In the central piazza, there's a fountain you can safely drink from, its cold water flowing via underground springs directly from the Aspromonte mountains.

In 1972, when I was five years old, I spent six months in Molochio with my mother, who had gone there to stay with my ailing grandfather. For many years, my *nonno* Alfonso had neglected a hernia, a simple condition that could have been treated with the right care. The day he died, everyone was calling his name to wake him. I walked in the room and said, "Can't you see that he has died already?" I was very close to my grandfather, and his death caused me great sadness; but even as a child, I felt that dealing with aging and death was something that I was supposed to do, that I had to take charge of the situation somehow.

Our neighbor in Molochio, Salvatore Caruso, was about the same age as my grandfather. In 2012, forty years after my grandfather's death, Salvatore and I would appear in the same issue of the scientific journal *Cell Metabolism* for my group's discovery that a low-protein diet, based on the eating habits of Molochio's elders, is associated with low cancer and overall mortality rates in the US population. The cover image of 108-year-old Salvatore standing among the Calabrian olive trees made the pages of *The Washington Post* and media around the globe. Two years after that, Salvatore was the oldest man in Italy, and one of four centenarians living in Molochio. Since there were only around two thousand people living there at the time, this meant Molochio had one of the highest proportions of centenarians in the world (four times that of Okinawa, Japan, which is believed to have the highest rate of centenarians for a large region).

Salvatore, who died in 2015 at the age of 110, started drinking from Molochio's fountain soon after he was born in 1905; given the exceptional longevity of so many of the town elders, it's tempting to think it might be the closest thing we have to a real fountain of youth. But while that's an interesting thought, I've spent most of my life studying the science of living long, and the truth is nothing so enchanted. You don't need to travel to Molochio to drink from its fountain of youth—but if you did, you would learn many of the secrets of longevity from its centenarians.

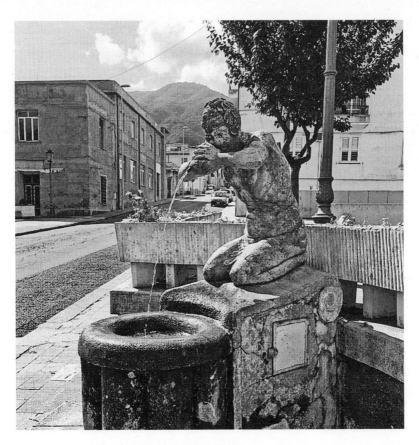

1.1. The fountain in the piazza of Molochio

From Tradition to Science

Whether by luck or destiny, my life took a path that has given me a unique and invaluable perspective on different diets and cultures. From the Calabrian diet of Molochio, where I spent childhood summers, to the pescetarian Ligurian diet of Genoa, where I was raised, to the heavy American diets of Chicago and Texas, to the health-obsessed diet of that mecca of youthfulness, Los Angeles—I've lived the full range of good, bad, and excellent nutrition, which has helped me formulate hypotheses about the connection between food, disease, and longevity. It also helped me realize that in order to understand how people can live long, healthy lives, we need to go beyond scientific, epidemiological, and clinical studies and investigate actual populations that age successfully.

Although I didn't know it at the time, I grew up between two places that boast among the healthiest traditional diets in the world. Unlike other regions of Italy famous for their meats (Tuscany) or their heavy cream-based sauces (Lazio, Emilia-Romagna), Liguria and Calabria maintained a cuisine based on complex carbohydrates and vegetables, with dishes like minestrone, *pansotti al sugo di noce* (a ravioli-like pasta with vegetable filling served in a walnut sauce), and *farinata* (garbanzo beans and olive oil). During the summers of my childhood in Calabria, we lived simply; almost every morning my brother or sister or I walked up the hill to the bakery to buy fresh bread, hot from the oven, dark from the whole wheat from which it was made. About once every other day, for either lunch or dinner, we ate *pasta e vaianeia*, which consisted of a small amount of pasta tossed together with large amounts of vegetables, particularly green beans cooked in the pod. Another common dish was *stoccafisso*, or stockfish—a dried cod similar to *baccala* but without the salt—served with a vegetable side dish. Other common ingredients of our diet growing up were black olives, olive oil, and lots of tomatoes, cucumbers, and green peppers. Meat was a once-a-week treat; only on Sundays would we have homemade *maccheroni* pasta with *polpette* (meatballs)—two each—or sometimes a small steak. The most common drinks were water (from the mountain spring), local wine, tea, coffee, and almond milk. We often drank goat's milk instead of cow's milk in the morning. Between meals we were allowed to snack only on peanuts, almonds, hazelnuts, walnuts, raisins, grapes, or corn on the cob. Once we finished dinner around 8 p.m., we usually wouldn't eat anything until the next morning. Even at our celebratory village fairs, the sweets were made with nuts and dried fruit. And instead of ice cream, we would often have *granita*, the frozen dessert somewhere between a smoothie and a sorbet. Made with lots of fruit, it is, in my opinion, the best dessert in the world, but it does contain a lot of sugar. We had to go six miles down the road, to the town of Taurianova, to find the good one.

The traditional diet of Genoa and its region Liguria is arguably *as* healthy as that of Calabria's; low in sugar, it consists of a lot of vegetables, garbanzo beans, olive oil, anchovies, codfish, and mussels, all of which represent important components of the Longevity Diet I present in this book.

From Ligurian to Chicagoan

When I was twelve years old, I would lock myself in my room with my electric guitar, turn the amplifier up to ten, and play along to the albums of Dire Straits, Jimi Hendrix, and Pink Floyd. I dreamed of going to America to become a rock star. That opportunity came in 1984 when, at age sixteen, I left Genoa to live with my aunt in Chicago. A music-crazed teenager, I arrived in the Little Italy district of Melrose Park, in the Chicago suburbs, with my guitar sticking out of my backpack, lugging a portable amp. My spoken-language skills were so bad that the immigration official stamped "no English" on my passport. Chicago had an incredible music scene. I took guitar lessons with Stewart Pearce, an iconic local bebop player. I was mostly interested in rock, but I knew that learning to play jazz and bebop would make me a much better rock guitar player. On weekends, I would sneak out of my aunt's house and take the L train downtown, where I would plug in and jam with musicians in blues clubs all night long.

My exposure to some of the best blues in the world coincided with my exposure to some of the unhealthiest food in the world—what I consider "the heart attack diet." At the time, I knew nothing about nutrition and aging, but I remember thinking something must be wrong with the Windy City diet because so many of my relatives there—mostly ethnic Calabrians—were dying of cardiovascular diseases, which were relatively uncommon in southern Italy in general, and were particularly rare in my extended family.

These southern Italians in America were eating bacon and sausage with eggs for breakfast, then lots of pasta, bread, and meat for lunch, often having meat again for dinner. They also consumed high quantities of cheese, milk, and high-fat, high-sugar desserts. The famous Chicago pizza had more calories from cheese than from the dough. Drinks were usually sodas or equally high-fructose fruit juices. To make matters worse, much of the food we Chicagoans ate was fried. Not surprisingly, many people I knew were overweight or obese by age thirty. Although I never became obese, I ate like everyone else and grew a lot during my three years in Chicago. My height shot up to six feet two, almost eight inches taller than my father and four inches taller than my brother. A possible explanation for this was all the meat suddenly in my diet, which, along with protein, probably contained steroid hormones.

I graduated high school in Chicago and headed south to study jazz performance at the famous University of North Texas College of Music. I could never have imagined eating more or becoming bigger than I was in Chicago—until I joined the Army Reserve as a way to pay for my education in Texas. Arriving for boot camp in Fort Knox, Kentucky, I joined a battalion of Army tankers who trained with the Marines and took pride in pushing themselves to the limit. We slept only three or four hours a night, did push-ups and other vigorous exercises all day long, and we ate—a lot.

I spent two summers at Fort Knox doing things I never would have believed myself capable of. It was the toughest and probably the best training of my life. The Army taught me how to get things done quickly, meeting the highest standards while minimizing or eliminating mistakes. Our trainers expected the impossible all the time. If you could do fifty push-ups, they told us, you should be going for a hundred. If you could run two miles in twelve minutes, they'd scream, you should finish in ten. I found out that sometimes when the impossible is expected, it can be achieved— eventually I was able to run two miles in ten minutes.

The Army diet was based on meat and carbohydrates, with sugary sodas allowed as a reward only if we had a combined run, push-up, and sit-up score of 200—which meant about seventy push-ups and sixty sit-ups in under two minutes each, plus running two miles in under ten and a half minutes. In retrospect,

I can see how addicted we all were to sugary drinks; we craved that mix of phosphoric acid, caramel coloring, and sugar, and everyone envied the very few who could reach that 200-point mark.

This diet, along with the grueling exercise regimen, made me a lot bigger, increasing the size of my muscles and making me stronger—at least that's what I assumed at the time. As I will explain in more detail in a later chapter, our recent studies indicate that a protein-rich diet, which can increase muscle size, may not necessarily translate into increased muscle strength and that a periodic low-protein, low-sugar diet, alternating with periods of normal protein intake, may do more to generate new muscle cells (which we currently think has more to do with strength than size does) while promoting health. In the ten years after basic training, during which my diet consisted of a lot of meat, fats, and proteins, my strength and stamina were dramatically reduced. But then I slowly switched to the Longevity Diet, and more than twenty-five years later I can do about the same number of push-ups and sit-ups as I did at boot camp when I was nineteen and supposedly in peak shape.

My stint in the Army eventually got me interested in how and why different types of diets can improve health without negatively affecting muscle mass and strength. The answer lies in nutritechnology, a new field I have helped create, in which we treat ingredients found in normal food as a complex set of molecules that, in specific doses and combinations, can have drug-like beneficial properties that we can harness to delay aging and prevent disease.[1]

In Tune with Evolution

My destination after finishing boot camp was Denton, Texas, just north of Dallas, home of the University of North Texas and one of the largest and best jazz performance programs in the world, where I was set to pursue an undergraduate degree in jazz performance. The program was tough, requiring an all-out, sixteen-hour-a-day, seven-days-a-week effort as a freshman. Jazz greats like pianist Dan Haerle and guitarist Jack Petersen became my teachers.

Many people in my career as a scientist who know about my beginnings as a jazz musician wonder how I came to make such a drastic change in my life's direction. The truth is, though music and science are obviously very different, you might be surprised at how much my musical training has helped me in the lab and spurred me on to discoveries that required creative approaches.

If you're trained from childhood to recognize chords, the ability to recognize frequencies and intervals isn't that difficult. It's like learning a new language, akin to a child recognizing spoken words and understanding what is being said. However, I was a mostly self-taught guitar player who learned through listening, so being all of a sudden exposed to a new language was particularly challenging for me; in the jazz program, I learned how to understand and write in a language I had always known simply as sound.

Similarly, as a scientist, you are always observing; but that observation is useless if you can't transform it into data or hypotheses. Musical training turned out to be essential for many of the discoveries I made about why we age and how it's connected to nutrition. When I started my research on aging, everyone could see that organisms aged, and everyone suspected that genes were somehow involved in that process; but the scientific community had no idea how to translate these observations into quantifiable genetic and molecular explanations. What were the harmonies and melodies of life and death? How could we decipher and transcribe these incredibly complex processes so that we might act upon and change them?

As an example of how my music training informed my scientific inquiry, here's one of my favorite analogies, which I use to explain what's missing from the prevalent "free radical" theory of aging, which holds that antioxidants alone (higher doses of vitamin C, for example) can extend the healthy human lifespan: Trying to extend your lifespan by increasing your intake of vitamin C is like trying to improve a Mozart symphony by increasing the number of cello players. The cello is a beautiful instrument, but to improve a Mozart symphony, you need to be a better composer than Mozart. Adding cellos alone won't do it. The healthy human lifespan is much more complex than a Mozart symphony. It took billions of years of evolution for it to reach the current state of near-perfection. We cannot expect a simple supplement to make something that's almost perfect even better, so we cannot expect that we will live healthier and longer lives just by drinking orange juice. Not surprisingly, supplementation with antioxidants has not even been shown to extend the lifespan of mice.

Another advantage musical studies gave me as a scientist was a training in improvisation and composition, important elements in jazz, to be sure, and also in science; improvisation challenges you to understand what you hear in relation to what you play so thoroughly and instantaneously that you can react to and match it on the fly. But this is only the start, since in jazz eventually the improvisation breaks free from the chord progression, often violating rules that would never be violated in classical music. However, the improviser is always aware of the chords, and the violation must follow new rules, albeit much more flexible ones. In science, this skill keeps you on the lookout for ideas that might be new or surprising but that are also well grounded, as opposed to looking for trendy discoveries that are just variations on previous breakthroughs. Composition instead forces you to write music that no one has written before; but unlike with improvisation, the music must be structured, and all the melodies and harmonies, as well as the instruments playing them and the way they are played, must be defined. In science and medicine, the music composer approach pushes you to look for new ideas, new hypotheses, but it also requires that the intervention has a mathematical foundation and is in harmony with the human body and its history. I call this being in tune with evolution. For example, as I will discuss elsewhere in the book, if we use a drug that lowers glucose, we are not considering the harmony of the human body, since that drug is disrupting a normal function of the organism. Although this may lead to a temporary solution (lower glucose), in the long run it will usually also lead to problems (adverse side effects). If instead we can rejuvenate the insulin-resistant muscle cells that cause the high glucose levels and render them more functional, we are making changes that maintain and even increase the harmony of the human body. Further, if this rejuvenation is activated by taking advantage of environments and conditions that echo our past and more ancient organisms, then we are not only taking advantage of the harmony, but we are also "in tune with evolution," since that process matches the "frequencies" of our history. Fasting, which is the focus of much of this book, activates coordinated responses that are in tune with evolution because starvation was encountered by all organisms, starting with bacteria, billions of years before *Homo sapiens* even existed. For this reason, it is clearly one of the most powerful interventions we can rediscover to promote coordinated changes that do not disrupt the harmony of the human body.

Without scientists and researchers thinking outside the box and being open to new possibilities and ideas, many of the greatest scientific and medical discoveries could never have been made—from Alexander Fleming's discovery of penicillin, to James Watson and Francis Crick and others' unraveling of the structure of DNA.

It was at the University of North Texas that I decided to switch my studies from music to science. One day during my second year there, an academic counselor asked me when I was going to enroll in Music Teaching, a course in which I would have to direct a marching band. It was the marching band that decided it. I had no intention of ever leading a marching band! For one thing, I was a rock musician. But for another, was this really what I wanted to do with my life? All of a sudden I didn't think so. I still play guitar to this day, but after a few days of wandering the streets of Denton, Texas, I decided that I wanted to devote my life to the study of how we age—or rather, how we might stay young and healthy for as long as possible.

I had noticed people I knew in their thirties worrying about "getting old." And it seemed like forty was the age at which people started to become vulnerable to major disease. As a twenty-year-old, I wondered: Why can't we push that back to fifty, sixty, even further? The field of aging provided a fantastic opportunity. It combined the impossible scientific task of understanding why we grow old and die with the idea I was just beginning to understand: that if we can effectively act on the aging process, we can postpone and even prevent many common diseases, enabling people to stay young and healthy as long as possible.

Along with my musical training, another element of my background has helped me in my career, and that is self-doubt. After making the decision to switch programs, I went to see the chairman of the biochemistry department, excited to discuss my new program of study. He was, to put it mildly, highly skeptical of a jazz performance major who had never taken a biology course, who now wanted to transfer into the biochemistry program to study aging. He told me that I was crazy and that I wouldn't last a semester. His reaction gave me pause—maybe he was right. My father was a policeman, and my mother, as was the cultural norm when I grew up, ran the house and only worked occasionally as a tailor; neither of my parents, who had emigrated to Genoa from the south, had more than a primary school education. So I wasn't sure I could do it. Maybe I was being presumptuous; maybe it was ridiculous to think that I'd be able to keep up. In retrospect, I realize it was probably this doubt that helped me succeed—in the program and as a scientist. My lab's motto and modus operandi is "paranoia." On the one hand, I teach my students never to trust their results, nor those of others, and always to expect that something will go wrong—the great result they might be so excited about will probably change under further scrutiny and experimentation, or when looked at from a different angle. On the other hand, I teach them that everything is possible. Think of big ideas; if you can dream it, you might be able to do it.

Our popular culture depicts scientists as confident-leader types, sure of what they're doing and the outcomes they will achieve. And it's true that this is a mind-set I frequently encounter at universities and in hospitals. Even in my college days, though, I understood that confidence was a way for arrogance to usurp knowledge. I believe the most revolutionary discoveries come from creativity and doubts because they first appear as crazy ideas, but then undergo a grueling process that makes them real and repeatable.

I didn't let my doubts stop me back then, and a year later I was thriving in the biochemistry program, working in the lab of the same doctor who had so doubted me. Soon I would be driving sixty miles a day to work in the lab of Dr. Robert Gracy, a leading aging research expert in Texas, where I would begin studying one of the most important aspects of aging: the process by which proteins are damaged. We can think of proteins as both the bricks that support an organism and the switchboard that transmits biological information from cell to cell, or within cells. For example, growth hormone is the protein that circulates in the blood-activating growth hormone receptors on the surface of cells, which promotes human growth. Like all proteins, growth hormone can be modified and damaged through aging, which can affect its function. Dr. Gracy's research group was studying how to potentially reverse this protein damage. This study would be the beginning of my research in the extraordinary field of longevity.

Hamburgers, french fries, and other unhealthy foods, especially Tex-Mex, remained my everyday diet throughout my undergraduate studies in Texas. Tex-Mex combines the worst food elements, transforming the relatively healthy Mexican cuisine into a terribly unhealthy one by frying everything and adding low-quality cheeses and meats. In spite of my new area of study, it didn't occur to me yet that my diet could affect my health and might be setting me up for disease. Not surprisingly, a few years after graduating from college, my cholesterol and blood pressure were high, and doctors were ready to load me up with statins and hypertension drugs. But by then I had joined the UCLA laboratory of Dr. Roy Walford, who was at the time the world's leading expert on nutrition and longevity. My diet, and life, were both about to change.

Chapter 2

Aging, Programmed Longevity, and Juventology

Why We Age

The approach in this book is different from that of the great majority of nutrition books because I focus on keeping organisms young, not treating individual diseases or conditions. So it's important to understand what aging is and the strategies that have the best chance of slowing it down without causing side effects.

"Aging" refers to the changes that occur over time to both organisms and objects. These changes aren't necessarily negative. In fact, although humans and most other organisms become dysfunctional in old age, growing older can actually bring improvements as well. For example, New York marathon winners are typically in their thirties, and many of the top finishers are in their forties. This suggests that there can be overall positive changes in the human body associated with aging.

So why do we age? Clearly every object around us, from houses to cars, gets old and deteriorates, so perhaps a better question is this: Why wouldn't humans and all other organisms also age and die?

Natural selection, the process Charles Darwin and Alfred Wallace described to explain evolution, has resulted in mechanisms that protect an organism, such as DNA repair, until it can generate healthy offspring. Over millions of years of evolution, the lifespan of an organism will tend to get longer if its ability to generate healthy offspring also increases. Both Wallace and Darwin also hypothesized that aging and death may be programmed so that organisms could age on purpose and die prematurely if it were advantageous to the species—to avoid overcrowding, for example. You can think of it like a company that establishes mandatory retirement at age sixty-five in order to allow younger employees to be hired, with the idea that ultimately this benefits the company. Both scientists abandoned this theory because, at the time, it would have been extremely difficult to demonstrate, since they did not have the computational, molecular biology, and genetics tools we have now.

A century and a half later, my laboratory produced one of the first pieces of experimental evidence for this "programmed aging" hypothesis. We showed that a selfish group of microorganisms—in this case baker's yeast that had been genetically manipulated to invest in their own protection and live as long as possible—would eventually become extinct, whereas shorter-lived microorganisms willing to sacrifice themselves and die early would seed future generations. In other words, the genetic alterations that make the organism act selfishly and live longer decrease its chances of generating healthy offspring. Whether human beings are actually programmed to die, however, has not been demonstrated.

To fully demonstrate programmed aging, one must first demonstrate group selection—one of the most hotly debated and challenged theories of evolutionary biology. Group selection posits that groups of organisms can act in an altruistic way, to protect or benefit the group at the individual's expense.

In most cases, it can be argued that altruistic behavior—a bird flying in front of the flock, for instance, thereby taking additional risks for the sake of the group—is just a case of paying one's dues, and that the risk taken will eventually benefit the individual taking the risk. But when an organism dies to benefit others, it's impossible to deem it a selfish act. Either death is occurring by chance (i.e., it serves no purpose), or it's programmed and altruistic. Over the past ten years, I have argued for programmed aging in a series of public debates against experts who argued for traditional evolutionary aging theories. After two such debates, in Texas and California, the audience, made up of scientists, was asked to vote on the theory that seemed right. In both cases I lost, though the vote and following discussions suggested I had convinced nearly half of them. Why? I believe it's because current evolutionary theories are accepted as dogma, and most scientists just aren't willing to consider alternative possibilities. To maximize the chance for everyone to make it to 110 healthy, it is important to consider these evolutionary theories and take advantage of the programs that have evolved to extend longevity in response to changes in the environment. For example, we showed that the "altruistic death program" described above is inactivated by starvation, indicating that an organism left without food no longer dies to benefit others, probably because the others are not expected to be around to benefit.

There are hundreds of theories of how and why we age. Many are partially true and overlap. For example, the popular free radical theory of aging I already mentioned proposes that oxygen and other reactive molecules that function as oxidants can cause damage to virtually all components of a cell and organism, similar to the rusting of metals when exposed to oxygen and water. Tom Kirkwood's "disposable soma" theory is another well-received theory of aging. It proposes that organisms invest in reproduction, in offspring and in themselves, but only to the level necessary to generate healthy offspring. The soma, our body—which is the carrier of the genetic material contained in our sperm cells and oocytes—is therefore disposable once it has generated a sufficient number of offspring. Unflattering as it sounds, under this theory we are merely disposable carriers of DNA.

Because these theories focus on the aging process and not on the potential for organisms to stay young, fifteen years ago I came up with my own explanation of aging: the "programmed longevity" theory.[1] I proposed that an organism could, in fact, afford a greater investment in self-protection against aging, and that this could have important implications for human life and the prevention of diseases; since by altering the "longevity program," we could postpone the age at which we begin to become frail and sick. Imagine, for example, moving this age from fifty to seventy. If this is possible, you might wonder, then why did this longevity program ever become dormant?

The answer is not that it is impossible to maximize both protection and reproduction, but that the level of current protection is sufficient to carry out the task. The other reason for the program to have remained dormant is that historically we reproduced, or tried to reproduce, much more frequently than we do now. So for the great majority of human history, activating a program that reroutes so much energy away from reproduction to use for protection and repair would not have been advantageous.

Consider this analogy: Would it be possible to build a plane that could fly years longer than current models without its performance suffering?

The answer is yes. There are at least two ways to accomplish this:

1. The longer-lived plane would need more fuel and more maintenance for each mile it flies to prevent damage.
2. The longer-lived plane would require superior technology to reduce damage while using the same amount of fuel and maintenance as current models.

Now let's apply this to humans:

1. People who live longer would need more energy to perform more maintenance (DNA repair, cellular regeneration, etc.).
2. People who live longer would need to get better at utilizing energy to increase protection against aging and maintaining normal function for longer.

However, there may be no evolutionary reason to do it, because for the human species to continue to thrive, aging and death at eighty is perfectly acceptable. But what if we wanted to be just a little more selfish and live an extra thirty healthy years? Is it possible to improve the protection and repair systems to stay young longer, or even become younger? Or have we reached a maximum level of protection?

I believe, and the data indicate, that we have not—that it is indeed possible to improve the body's protective systems or make these systems continue to work longer so that we undergo decline and begin to encounter diseases not at age forty to fifty but at age sixty to seventy or better yet, never encounter many of them at all. In the following chapters I will show how genetic or dietary interventions can not only delay diseases but actually *eliminate* a major portion of chronic diseases in mice, monkeys, and even humans to extend longevity. At the foundation of these effects is what I called programmed longevity: a biological strategy to influence longevity and health through cellular protection and regeneration to stay younger longer.

Juventology

Discussions about theories of aging are great entertainment for scientists but not much use to anyone else. Under the programmed longevity theory, how and why we age is not as interesting as how we stay young. Because of the importance of this distinction, I coined a term for this area of inquiry: "juventology," the study of youth. What's the difference? A great deal.

If you are trying to understand why a car ages, you might study the engine and conclude that over time it slowly rusts. To make it last longer, you might add an antioxidant additive to the fuel or motor oil. This is essentially what the free radical theory of aging supports as a way to extend healthy longevity. But this is like what I said before about vitamin C and the Mozart symphony: you can't improve Mozart's compositions by just adding cellos—you have to write a better symphony. But for the sake of argument, let's suppose that you could slow the aging of the engine a little by adding a lot of antioxidants. This aging process and the small effect of the antioxidants on it becomes irrelevant, however, if the owner of the car rebuilds the engine every ten years, replacing the damaged parts with brand-new ones.

The same applies to the human body: we can try to understand how it ages and attempt to slow that down, or we can identify ways to eliminate aged components and periodically replace them with young ones. In this case, it doesn't matter how the body ages, whether by oxidation or some other mechanism. The goal changes from protecting the body from damage to improving protection and, more importantly, repair and replacement/regeneration.

In both cases the body ages with time, but if we can program health to last longer, the system will trigger protection, repair, and replacement mechanisms to maintain the organism's vigor and functionality. This is the difference between the current gerontology/aging-based approach and what I think is a more effective juventology-based approach. It is worth keeping in mind that protecting the body from aging and damage is also important because we are a long way from being able to repair and replace molecules, cells, and systems perfectly. Thus, combining the gerontology and juventology approaches is ideal.

Throughout this book, I will describe specific dietary changes that have protective, regenerating, and rejuvenating effects. As my laboratory has discovered, there is a clear connection between nutrients and longevity genes, which can be activated to promote cellular reprogramming and regeneration so that an organism can stay healthy longer and, as a consequence, maximize what we call "healthspan," or healthy lifespan.

The Discovery of the Aging Genes and Networks

To keep organisms young, we must "reprogram" the "youth period" from a forty-to-fifty-year length to a sixty-to-seventy-year program or longer. To learn how to reprogram longevity though, I had to better understand its molecular mechanisms. The dietary interventions described later in the book are based on discoveries made in part by my laboratory's research into just this.

In 1992, I came to UCLA, at that time one of the world's leading centers of longevity research, to devote myself to the genetics and biochemistry of longevity. I had put my career as a rock guitarist on hold, though I did perform in Los Angeles and toured on the West Coast during my first three years of graduate school. Perhaps influenced by the Hollywood obsession with staying eternally young, each of the two rival research universities of the City of Angels had attracted its own master in the field of aging: famous pathologist Roy Walford was at UCLA, and renowned neurobiologist Caleb Finch was at USC.

I elected to join Walford's group for my doctoral work. Under his watch, I studied the effect of caloric restriction—how reducing the daily calories consumed by mice and men by 30 percent every day affects their aging and lifespan. However, Roy and I spoke only via video conference because he had decided to lock himself away for two years, along with seven other people, in a sealed environment in the middle of the Arizona desert. Called Biosphere 2, this self-imposed exile was an experiment to understand whether and how humans could survive in a completely sealed environment, producing all the food they needed: a useful experiment in the responses of humans to a highly regulated environment with possible applications for living on space stations. I went to Arizona at the end of the two years to welcome the eight adventurers as they came out of Biosphere 2. As part of the experiment, they had been calorie restricted and consumed very few calories a day for two years. When they emerged at the end of it, they were extremely thin and looked angry.

After being in Walford's UCLA lab for two years, I still had little insight into the secrets of aging. Mice were too complex to allow rapid identification of the genes that regulate and affect aging. Also seeing the angry faces of the Biospherians made me think that there must be a better way than chronic calorie restriction to delay aging, and I was impatient to find it. It prompted me to move to the biochemistry department, and the laboratory of Joan Valentine and Edith Gralla, to study aging in baker's yeast: a simple unicellular organism that allowed me to study the molecular foundation for life, aging, and death.

We think of yeast as an ingredient in bread and beer, but *Saccharomyces cerevisiae* (baker's yeast) is in fact one of the most studied organisms in science. This single-cell organism is inexpensive to work with and easy to study. It is so easy to work with that some scientists carry out yeast experiments at home. It's also

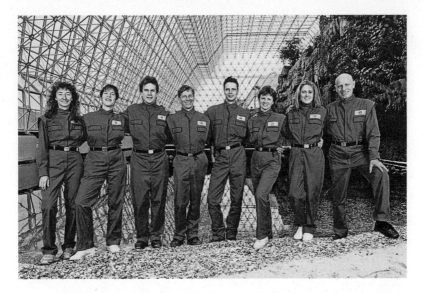

2.1. *Roy Walford (far right) and the Biospherians at the beginning of the experiment, 1991*

easy to modify genetically, by simply removing or adding one or more of its roughly six thousand genes.

A small group of scientists, including myself at UCLA and Brian Kennedy at MIT, decided the easiest way to understand how humans age is to identify the genes that regulate the aging of simple organisms, like yeast, and eventually move back to mice and humans. There was a big risk, however: What if our discoveries about how yeast ages had no relevance to humans? Most scientists studying aging in mice and humans had assumed that to be the case and were not that interested in our research on these very simple organisms.

But I had faith it would work and was determined to try; the risk was big but the potential payoff—figuring out the molecular mechanisms of aging—was worth it. My first step was to define a new scientific approach to studying aging. Because aging in yeast was studied only by a method called "replicative aging," which would be equivalent to studying human aging by determining the maximum number of children a woman could have, I developed a method called "yeast chronological life" and used it to identify a set of genes important to aging. This method allowed me to measure aging chronologically—in other words, the same way we measure it for humans or mice—by being able to monitor every few days how many of these microorganisms remained alive. It was 1994, and no one had ever identified a gene that regulated the aging process in any organism. Thanks to the work of Thomas Johnson at the University of Colorado and Cynthia Kenyon at UC San Francisco, it was known that genes could make worms live longer—just not what genes they were or how they worked.

With three Nobel laureates and seven members of the National Academy of Sciences in the pharmacology and biochemistry departments, UCLA was science heaven. I was surrounded by great geneticists, biochemists, and molecular biologists, all ready to help. I didn't even have to knock, because the doors—even those of the Nobelists—were almost always open.

Even so, we didn't tell people we were working on aging. Although within ten to fifteen years the field would explode, back then it was considered a strange, even crazy area of study, and we were considered an odd group. When people asked what I was working on, I would say, "Free radical biochemistry."

After just one year I made two important discoveries using the method I had invented:

1. If I starved yeast—by removing all the nutrients available to them and giving them only water—they lived twice as long.

2. Sugar is one of the nutrients responsible for yeast aging fast and dying early. It activates two genes, RAS and PKA, that are known to accelerate aging, and it inactivates factors and enzymes that protect against oxidation and other types of damage.

In a short period in the biochemistry department, I had identified not only the first gene regulating the aging process but also the entire signaling pathway, all thanks to a very simple organism.

The system was so simple and so new that the scientific community was in disbelief and struggled to understand, let alone accept, the chronological aging system and the discovery of the pro-aging sugar pathway. Leading science journals refused to publish the findings my mentors and I found so extraordinary, so I used the discoveries as the basis for my doctoral thesis, as well as two other publications, which were ignored for several years.

It wasn't until 1996 that anyone showed any interest in my discovery. The leading aging research at the time was being done on worms, and Tom Johnson, who was trying to identify an unknown gene that made worms live longer, invited me to present my data on the "sugar pathway" at a conference. When my presentation ended, the room was absolutely silent. The stars of the aging field, who years later would become my colleagues and friends, stared at me as if I had grown horns—no one had ever heard of the system I was working with (yeast chronological aging), nor of the genes I had identified, and anyway, very few believed that similar genes and strategies could be affecting aging in such different organisms.

A few years later, encouraged by continuing to discover similarities between my findings in yeast and those of the teams

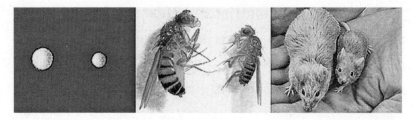

2.2. Yeast, fruit flies, and dwarf mice with similar mutations in growth genes all have record longevity.

studying worms, which now included Gary Ruvkun at Harvard, I published an article proposing that many if not all organisms age in similar ways and that the genes and "molecular strategy" to achieve longer lifespans would be similar or the same in yeast, worms, mice, and, yes, humans.[2] This was heresy, and the great majority of scientists dismissed it as a crazy idea with no relevance to human aging, since it was based on discoveries made in a microorganism.

It would take another six years for our data on genes activated by sugars to get published, along with the discovery of the pro-aging genes activated by amino acids and proteins (see fig. 2.2).[3] Eight more years passed before different laboratories would confirm these data experimentally in mice, and another ten years before my own lab provided initial evidence that similar genes and pathways may protect humans against age-related diseases.[4]

Knowing that "dwarf yeast" with longevity mutations in the growth genes (TOR-S6K) could live up to five times longer than normal yeast, and that "dwarf flies and mice" with similar genetic mutations could live up to twice as long as normal mice, in 2006

I started research on the human version of the growth gene known to correlate to record longevity in mice (see fig. 2.2). Through my colleague Pinchas Cohen, who is now dean of the USC Leonard Davis School of Gerontology, I learned of the work of Jaime Guevara-Aguirre, an endocrinologist who had spent decades studying a community of extremely short people in Ecuador who lacked the receptor for growth hormone, a disorder known as Laron syndrome. After five years of working together, we published our findings concluding that there was a major decrease in the incidence of cancer and diabetes in subjects with Laron syndrome (see fig. 2.4), despite poor diet (consuming large quantities of fried food) and unhealthy lifestyle choices (smoking, drinking, etc.).[5] Our finding made this group of short individuals from remote villages in Ecuador famous around the world—everyone wanted to hear about this group of little people who appeared to hold the secret that could protect everyone from cancer, diabetes, and possibly other diseases. We were even invited to present our research to the Pope, accompanied by one of our Laron subjects. Journalists described these people as being free from disease. "It doesn't matter what we eat," the Laron subjects told reporters, "because we are immune from diseases." Of course, this is not the case; a few have developed both cancer and diabetes, but these diseases occur rarely, and much less frequently than they appear in their non-Laron relatives living in the same houses and consuming the same food. Recently, we also published our studies on the brain function of this Laron group and concluded that they have cognitive function that is typical of younger individuals.[6] In other words, their brains appear to be younger than they are,

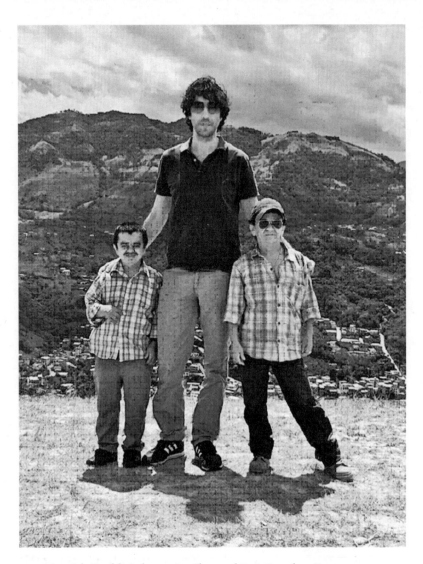

2.3. *Me with Freddi Salazar Aguilar and Luis Sanchez Romero (both with Laron mutations) in their native Ecuador*

which is in agreement with the findings published by the Andrzej Bartke laboratory in mice with similar mutations.[7] After these studies and many trips to Ecuador, the country, particularly the isolated Andes to the south, became a magical place for me, and

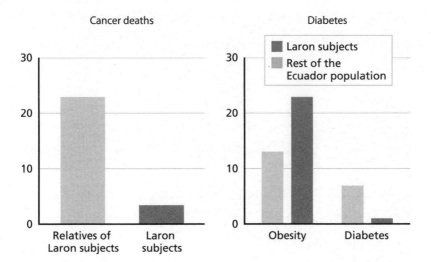

2.4. *Individuals with mutations in the growth hormone receptor are protected from disease.*

I go back as often as possible. Jaime and I argue all the time, but we continue to work very closely and have forged a fruitful friendship.

These findings were the last missing pieces to support my theory that similar genes and longevity programs can protect organisms, ranging from simple ones such as yeast to complex ones like humans, against aging and disease. These alternative programs, such as those found in the Laron people, have probably evolved to deal with periods of starvation by minimizing growth and aging, while also stimulating regeneration. The mutation in the growth hormone receptor gene that these Ecuadorians carry appears to force the body to enter and stay in an "alternative longevity program" characterized by high protection, regeneration, and low incidence of disease. The rest of the book takes advantage of this genetic knowledge to identify everyday diets and a periodic fasting-mimicking diet that can regulate genes that protect against aging and diseases.

Connecting Nutrients, Genes, Aging, and Diseases

A risk factor is something that affects the probability of dying from or developing a particular disease. For example, obesity is a well-established risk factor for diabetes: it can increase by fivefold the chance of developing the disease. We think of poor nutrition, lack of exercise, and the genes we inherit from our parents as the major risk factors for diseases. But, by monitoring the age at which people are diagnosed with different diseases, we know that aging itself is the main risk factor for cancer, cardiovascular disease, Alzheimer's, and many other diseases. According to recent data, the probability that a twenty-year-old woman will develop breast cancer within the next ten years of her life is roughly 1 in 2,000. The risk is 1 in 24 for a seventy-year-old woman—that's an increase by almost a factor of 100.

As I have stated, my approach is different from that of almost all other nutrition books, in that my program doesn't focus on achieving a healthy weight or on any one specific disease independently of the long-term consequences of a treatment. If aging is the central risk factor for all major diseases, it's much smarter to intervene on aging itself than to try to prevent and treat diseases one by one. Even great success against one disease may be minimal or rendered irrelevant if accompanied by an increased incidence of another—few people know, for example, that curing cancer or cardiac disease today would increase the average lifespan by only a little over three years.

The lifespan of a mouse is about two and a half years, and tumors begin to appear in mice at the age of one and a half. People live on average more than eighty years, and most tumors begin to appear after age fifty. In relative terms, that is a similar proportion of life. Therefore, we can reduce the risk of cancer and many other diseases by acting on the longevity program, and we now know that we can do this through diet.

Figure 2.5 shows how sugars and proteins (amino acids) affect key genes and pathways widely recognized to accelerate aging: TOR-S6K, PKA, RAS, and IGF-1. To maximize and reprogram longevity in the human body, we need to continue to study how different diets control these genes and then apply the longevity program to all the diseases associated with aging. (See chapters 7 to 11 for disease-specific applications.) Clearly our strategy of studying the genetics and molecular biology of longevity in sim-

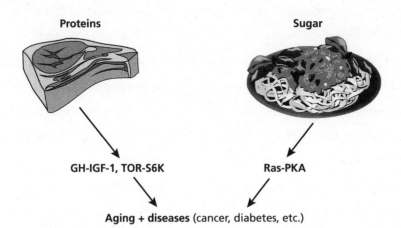

2.5. *The regulation of aging and diseases by sugar- and protein-activated pathways*

ple organisms paid off, though it took many years of hard work by groups made up of mostly geneticists and molecular biologists at universities all over the world.

From Studying Aging to Solving Medical Problems

After studying aging, my second passion, developed while working with Walford's group at UCLA, is using the biochemistry of longevity to solve medical problems. To optimize disease prevention and treatment, we need to know what causes disease at the molecular and cellular level and to understand how we can return those molecules and cells to their youthful, fully functioning states. To attempt to treat a disease without this information is like trying to fix a car without knowing how its engine or electrical system works. Repairing cars and planes is, of course, much simpler than repairing a sick human body.

Although this is a generalization, much of medical research is based on identifying drugs that can target a specific problem associated with a disease. For example, to treat cancer, researchers developed chemotherapy and other more specific drugs that preferentially kill cancer cells; to treat multiple sclerosis and other autoimmune diseases, scientists identified proteins and drugs that reduce the activity of specific immune cell populations or the inflammatory factors they generate. I argue that this is an incomplete approach that is not "in tune with evolution" and that would greatly benefit from being combined with, and in some cases replaced by, a "longevity-based" approach, preferably one awakening a program already present in the human body, once this is further demonstrated to be effective. For example, by starving a mouse receiving chemotherapy or other targeted therapies, we protect normal cells and organs while making the therapy more toxic to cancer cells (see chapter 7); and by applying cycles of a fasting-mimicking diet to a mouse with an autoimmune disease, we reduce the number of autoimmune cells while also activating regeneration of the damaged tissues (see chapter 11). Preliminary results indicate that these strategies may also be effective in humans.

While I was a research scientist working at USC, I had the opportunity to meet with children being treated for cancer at Children's Hospital Los Angeles. Italian researcher Lizzia Raffaghello, at the time a visiting scholar in Los Angeles, was puzzled by our effort to find ways to help people live longer and healthier lives to age one hundred and beyond, when her ward was full of children who might not make it to ten.

One of these patients was a girl from southern Italy. We considered isolating her neuroblastoma cells in the laboratory, to study them and understand what therapy might work best. But we came up against the hard reality that this type of study was not allowed by the hospital or by my department. The girl eventually returned to Italy, and sadly she died. I will never forget how she kept close watch on the intravenous saline solution bag, with the seriousness and maturity of a nurse ensuring a procedure is being carried out correctly.

Because of the impact that girl and the other sick children I'd met had on my vision of research, I decided to divide my lab between two areas of interest and two different missions. One team of researchers would continue to work on the biochemistry and genetics of aging; the other would work to solve medical problems using strategies based on our understanding of cellular protection, repair, and regeneration with an eye toward solutions that were inexpensive and could rapidly be translated into improved therapies. Because diet-based therapies do not involve new drugs, they can move through the Food and Drug Administration approval process quickly, and in some cases can be combined with standard-of-care drug-based therapies without FDA approval. From this effort came our discoveries of differential stress resistance and sensitization, which use prolonged fasting to push normal cells into a highly protected state while making cancer cells highly vulnerable to chemotherapy and other cancer therapies (see chapter 7). Other dietary strategies applicable to diabetes as well as autoimmune, cardiovascular, and neurodegenerative disorders also came from our effort to identify simple but powerful therapies for complex problems. But before we get to the diet itself, I'll explain how I've harnessed thirty years of research, both mine and that of other labs, to identify daily diets as well as periodic fasting-mimicking diets with the potential to extend healthy human longevity.

Chapter 3

The Five Pillars

The Longevity Revolution

Most popular diets and the experts behind them fail to take into consideration the most important reason to adopt a diet in the first place: living to a very old age and "dying healthy." We are so used to associating death with cancer, heart disease, or another illness that the concept of "dying healthy" seems alien. But this is the promise of the "longevity revolution."[1] Indeed, the concept is now strongly supported by experiments in simple organisms, mice, rats, monkeys, and humans. Based on biogerontology (study of the biology of aging), preventive medicine, and longevity research, we now know that the later years of life, even when life is extended, need not be associated with poor health and disease.

For example, the mice and rats we treat in the lab with different longevity diets live up to 40 percent longer *and* have far fewer diseases despite their longer lifespan compared to mice on standard diets. Long-term studies of monkeys on a calorie-restricted diet demonstrate a major reduction in disease incidence as well as lifespan extension. This is consistent with our recent study associating high protein intake with cancer and mortality in humans. In addition, we discovered that, as with the long-lived mice lacking growth hormone receptors, the Ecuadorian people with the same deficiency in the GH receptor rarely develop either diabetes or cancer and appear to be protected from age-dependent cognitive decline and possibly other diseases. Thus, dietary interventions that affect particular genes or genetic changes in those genes directly can extend not only longevity but healthy longevity in mice, primates, and humans. According to these studies, a precise Longevity Diet accompanied by periodic fasting-mimicking diets (which I describe in chapters 4 and 6, respectively) can, by regulating the set of "longevity genes," extend the healthy lifespan.

I've been lucky to see this kind of healthy longevity with my own eyes. In the past ten years, I was able to make many visits to the two oldest people in Italy: Salvatore Caruso, 110, and Emma Morano, 117, who have both now passed away. Emma was also the oldest living person in the world, and the oldest ever in Italy's recorded history. Both retained good memory skills, engaged in many activities on their own into old age, and were remarkable examples of healthy longevity. Emma exemplifies the importance of genetics on longevity (her diet wasn't particularly healthy), whereas Salvatore shows the influence of diet on human health. Thus, the study of people and populations with record longevity represents one of the key pillars I have used to identify the Longevity Diet described in this book.

Who Do You Listen To?

Among the longevity factors within your control, what you eat is the primary choice you can make that will affect whether you live to 60, 80, 100, or 110—and more important, whether you will get there in good health. So when it comes to dietary recommendations, it's crucial to listen to the right people. In an Internet-centered world, perhaps the most dangerous development for your health is the chaos generated by the idea that everyone can give dietary advice. It is essential to determine whether a so-called diet expert has the appropriate range of knowledge before deciding whether he or she is qualified to give you dietary advice.

On a recent train ride from Milan to Genoa, I had one of many entertaining experiences underlining that everyone believes themselves to be a diet expert. An old building administrator from Genoa explained how his wife's omelets were the key to maintaining his weight and health. The woman next to him protested that eggs have high cholesterol and that her pasta and zucchini were much healthier. When five such "dietary experts" had made their recommendations, they wondered why I had not jumped in.

"I think you'd better cut down on the number of fried eggs per week," I told the retired administrator.

"You know, I don't think I like you," he replied.

Because everyone eats, everyone feels he or she knows enough about food and health to give advice. Recently a woman asked me what I thought she and her son should eat to stay healthy. After hearing my advice, she responded, "I think the best thing to do is to eat everything in moderation."

I asked her, "Would you fly on an airplane that you had personally designed?"

She knew the correct answer to that question was absolutely not. Most planes are designed by teams of world-class engineers working at major aviation companies like Boeing and Airbus, using technology and insights going back to the Wright brothers and even Leonardo da Vinci. Why would you be willing to make key decisions that affect whether you and your loved ones will get cancer, diabetes, cardiovascular disease, and many other illnesses based on the silly idea that one should "eat in moderation"? What does that even mean?

In the class I teach on nutrition and longevity at USC, I ask my students how many calories there are in a bagel. Most think it's around 100 or 150 calories. In fact, most bagels provide between 250 and 500 calories, without cream cheese. When I started directing clinical trials in which participants are told exactly what to eat, I discovered that most people have no idea what it means to eat 0.36 grams of protein per pound of body weight per day. Even experienced health journalists have told me, "I wasn't sure if you meant that I should eat fifty grams of protein or fifty grams of food that contains proteins per day."

I mean protein, not food that contains protein. This minor misunderstanding alone could cause someone to become malnourished or sick—50 grams of garbanzo beans contains only 5 grams of protein, just 10 percent of what adults need to stay healthy.

I have also learned that "moderation" is relative. Consider the following daily menu: a glass of milk, two eggs and bacon, a small steak, a slice of cheese, some carrots, some pasta, a chicken filet, a salad with ranch dressing, a piece of cake, and two soft drinks. To many people, this represents eating in moderation. Yet this is the type of diet that has made the United States one of the world leaders in obesity and related diseases. The key to adopting a longevity diet is finding books, like this one, written by scientists or clinicians who have mastered as many of the Pillars of Longevity as possible. Although most healthy people will be able to make these dietary changes on their own, I do recommend if at all possible that you consult with a qualified medical doctor or registered dietitian, at least initially, and especially if you have food allergies and might need help personalizing the diet to your needs. You already bought this book, so you're on the right track.

As I have said, I based the great majority of dietary recommendations in this book not on my opinion, but on the Five Pillars of Longevity and the solid, consistent, scientific, and clinical evidence they provide. I don't talk about "miracle diets" or "cures," and I stay away from fad diets promising weight loss. Changing your diet to gear it toward healthy longevity will take some work. But it will be much easier than you imagine, and in many cases it will be more beneficial than drug therapies when you factor in both efficacy and side effects. Not to mention saving money on doctors and medications. In the long run, the life-extending benefits will be well worth the effort.

I'm confident in these claims because of the positive results achieved by thousands of people I have studied—either personally or through basic research, clinical trials, and genetic and epidemiological studies. I'm also confident because most of my recommendations for everyday diets match the diets of the very-long-lived populations that I, and other experts like Craig Wilcox in Okinawa, have studied. These individuals are concentrated in "blue zones," a term coined by Michel Poulain and Gianni Pes, and made popular by author Dan Buettner, to identify longevity hot spots, where diet and physical activity levels are believed to be a key factor in successful longevity. This book also takes into account dietary habits that were common in our history. For example, my disease-treatment recommendations in the later chapters of this book, specifically the fasting and fasting-mimicking diets, are based on scientific and clinical studies; but many of these interventions find echoes in ancient practices, such as religious fasting. Historically religious fasting was not adopted to prevent or treat disease but, since it was common for our ancestors and has now been tested on thousands of people, we know it to be generally feasible and safe.

The Five Pillars of Longevity

Most people are discouraged and often confused by nutritional news. Nutrient groups (fats, proteins, and carbohydrates) and also specific foods like eggs and coffee have all been described in scientific journals and the media as both good and bad for you. How do you decide what's right for you and your health? In fact, proteins, fats, and carbohydrates can be considered both good and bad for you depending on type and consumption. For example, proteins are essential for normal function, yet high levels of proteins, and particularly those from red meat and other animal sources, have been associated with increased incidence of several diseases. So we need a better system to filter out the noise and extract beneficial dietary information.

This is why I formulated the "Five Pillars of Longevity." This method is based on my own studies and also on the studies of many other laboratories and clinicians. It uses five research areas to determine whether a nutrient or combination of nutrients is good or bad for health and to identify the ideal combination of foods for optimal longevity.

I believe that many popular strategies and diets are inappropriate or only partially correct because they are based on just one or two pillars. This is important because while one nutrient may be protective against one condition or disease, it can negatively affect another, or it can protect middle-age individuals but hurt the very young or the elderly. An example: In adults age seventy and below, eating a relatively high-calorie diet will in most cases lead to weight gain and an increase in the risk for developing certain diseases. Yet in individuals over age seventy, the same diet and the consequent moderate weight gain can be protective against certain diseases and overall mortality. This is why it is important to follow the advice of someone who has an in-depth understanding of the complex relationship between nutrition, aging, and disease.

The Five Pillars of Longevity create a strong foundation for dietary recommendations and a filtering system to evaluate thousands of studies related to aging and disease, while also minimizing the burden of dietary change. When dietary choices are based on all the Five Pillars, they are unlikely to be contradicted or undergo major alterations as a consequence of new findings.

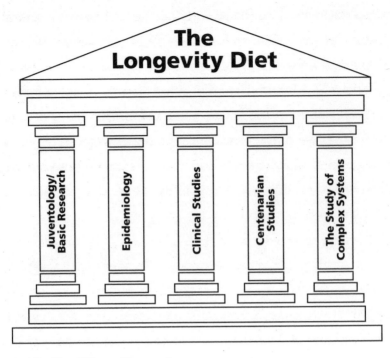

3.1. *The Five Pillars of Longevity*

THE FIVE PILLARS OF LONGEVITY:

■ **Basic/juventology research.** Without understanding how nutrients—such as proteins and sugars—affect cellular function, aging, age-dependent damage, and regeneration, it is difficult to determine the type and quantity of nutrients needed to optimize healthy longevity. Without animal studies to determine whether a diet can in fact extend longevity, in addition to having acute effects on general health, it is difficult to translate the basic discoveries to human interventions. As I mentioned earlier, I first started working with mice and humans in Walford's lab, but I soon discovered that a far simpler unicellular organism, yeast, could help us identify the fundamental properties of organisms. These could then be applied to humans, furnishing information related to molecular aspects of longevity—in particular, the ones linked to evolutionary principles. Using yeast, we were able to generate the differential stress resistance and sensitization theories that served as the foundation for a number of clinical trials testing the effect of fasting-mimicking diets in combination with cancer therapies. This basic/juventology research is where every one of our studies begins.

- **Epidemiology.** This is the study of the causes and important risk factors for disease and other health-related conditions in defined populations. Studying population-based risk factors is crucial to testing hypotheses generated by basic research. For example, if you hypothesize that excess sugar promotes abdominal fat storage and resistance to insulin, epidemiological research should confirm that people who consume high quantities of sugars have a high waist circumference and an increased risk for diabetes. After my initial focus on the genetics of aging and juventology, I carried out epidemiological studies related to aging and diseases, which taught me the tremendous value of understanding the health consequences of behavior in large populations.

- **Clinical studies.** Hypotheses formulated in basic and epidemiological studies eventually must be tested in randomized, controlled clinical trials. This is the gold standard to demonstrate efficacy. For example, a group of pre-diabetic subjects would be instructed to consume fewer sugars but otherwise maintain the same diet and calorie intake as before. The control group would be asked to maintain the same diet or reduce the intake of fat to match the calorie reduction in the reduced-sugar group. Understanding the importance of this pillar grew out of my own randomized clinical trials, and those of many others, testing the effect of a particular dietary component on risk factors for disease, such as cholesterol or fasting glucose levels, but also on a disease itself, such as cardiovascular disease.

- **Centenarian studies.** Once the data from basic/juventology, epidemiological, and clinical studies are available, there is still uncertainty about whether a specific diet or nutritional indication is in fact safe and beneficial after long-term use, and whether it is palatable enough for people not just to adopt it but to stick with it for the rest of their lives. Studies of various centenarian populations from around the world provide long-term evidence of the safety, efficacy, and compliance associated with a particular diet (for example, a low-sugar diet). To generate data for the fourth pillar, I have studied long-lived populations in Ecuador and southern Italy and consulted the work of my colleagues focusing on other very long-lived populations in high-longevity zones around the world.

- **Studies of complex systems.** This pillar is the result of my fascination with reductionism, physics, and the need to simplify the human body's complexity by identifying machines that can serve as models to teach us about the function and loss of function of human organs and systems. This last pillar can complement the others by providing reference points and useful analogies. For example, above I discuss how sugars can lead to disease. But sugars are also the most important nutrient for the human body. Sugar is to the body what gasoline is to a car—the central source of energy. So sugar is not the problem. It's the intake of excessive quantities of sugar, in combination with proteins and certain types of fats, that contributes to disease both directly and indirectly—by activating aging-related genes, creating insulin resistance, and triggering hyperglycemia. This last pillar furthers the analysis of a human problem by taking an engineering approach to generate a relatively simple model to understand the complex interactions between food, cellular damage, and aging.

Applying the Five Pillars of Longevity

As an example of how to apply the Five Pillars to analyze a diet's efficacy, let's examine the very popular high-protein, high-fat, and low-carb diet, such as the Atkins and Dukan diets. Should you go on this diet just because an "expert" told you that a small clinical trial or even a large epidemiological study shows that it causes weight loss and may lower cholesterol? The answer is definitely not, since when you analyze these diets, they are often based on just one or two pillars, rarely taking into account the entire foundation needed to support the selection of a diet that will optimize health and longevity. These are the diets that tend to get debunked over time. When you look at multidisciplinary studies, you realize that the high-protein, high-saturated-fat, and low-carb diet is one of the worst for your health. Populations with record longevity do not eat this way, and theoretical, clinical, and epidemiological studies supporting this kind of diet's long-term and longevity benefits are very few. Also, if we examine the laboratory studies, we see that both high protein intake and high saturated fat intake are associated with aging and disease, an additional and key vote against a high-protein, high-saturated-fat diet.

As you can see, even when a diet is touted as having been clinically studied, it doesn't mean that it has been studied as rigorously as necessary, so it is always wise to hesitate before adopting a new diet, and to look into how many of the Five Pillars it is based on. As we have shown in both our human and mouse studies, one diet fits most but does not fit all, and the levels of some dietary components must be modified depending on a person's age and physical state and based on his or her genes. In my laboratory, we treat food as a complex mixture of molecules—each capable of causing remarkable changes in your body, which is its own complex mixture of molecules.

If it already sounds confusing or difficult to follow, don't worry, I will make it as simple as possible in chapter 4.

Chapter 4

The Longevity Diet

You Are What You Eat

We all know the saying "You are what you eat." For most people, that translates to "avoid junk food." But this popular expression reflects a deeper truth. The food you eat can determine how you look and function, whether you sleep well at night, whether you will stay thin or gain weight, and whether your body shape is more like a pear or an apple. The type of food you eat determines whether your brain will use glucose or ketone bodies to obtain energy; and if you're a woman, the type and quantity of food you eat can affect your chances of becoming pregnant. It's important to eat food you truly enjoy, but it's also important to eliminate or minimize the consumption of food that will make your life shorter and sicker, and to increase the consumption of nutrients that will make your life longer and healthier.

Many ingredients aren't just food; they're actually molecules causing remarkable changes in the body—changes in their levels and combinations can reprogram the function of our cells and organs. As mentioned earlier, I call the understanding and use of food combinations to control these changes "nutritechnology." In this chapter, I will describe briefly what these ingredients are and what they do. Then I will explain their role in aging and disease, based on evidence using the Five Pillars of Longevity. I will also focus on the enjoyability of food—an important consideration that can determine how likely someone is to continue with a certain diet.

Proteins, Carbohydrates, Fats, and Micronutrients

There are three major components—what we call macronutrients—in the food we eat.

1. **Proteins** are generally composed of twenty amino acids, whose sequence determines their particular function. For example, a 3-ounce steak contains approximately 25 grams of protein. One of the most abundant proteins in meat is actin, which is involved in muscle contraction and many other cellular functions. After meat is eaten, the digestive system breaks it down into protein and then into amino acids. These amino acids are released first in the stomach and subsequently in the intestine. They are absorbed into the blood-

stream as single amino acids or chains of multiple amino acids. Eventually, amino acids are distributed to different cell types throughout the body, where they are used to generate new proteins, including the actin found in human muscle.

2. **Carbohydrates** are found in most foods you eat, either in their simple form (the sugars in fruit juices, honey, candy, or soft drinks) or in their complex form (the large chains of glucose and other sugars contained in vegetables or grains). Simple sugar can enter circulation immediately, increase blood glucose levels, and trigger the rapid release of insulin by the pancreas. Complex carbohydrates must be separated from other components in food and broken down into simple sugars before they can be absorbed by the body.

   When analyzing a food's nutritional value in terms of its carbohydrates and their quality, there are a couple of different measures. You've probably heard the terms "glycemic index" and "glycemic load." Glycemic index refers to the effect of a particular food on the levels of blood glucose. Orange juice has a glycemic index of about 50; white bread has an index of 95; a pure glucose drink has an index of 100. However, glycemic index assumes that you are eating a standard portion of carbohydrates. Glycemic *load* is a more useful measurement because it reveals information about both the characteristics of a specific carbohydrate *and* its quantity. For example, whole-wheat bread has a high glycemic index (71) but a slice of whole bread has a relatively low glycemic load (9). Compare that to sponge cake, with its relatively low glycemic index (46) but higher glycemic load (17). You should be more concerned about the glycemic load, since it takes into account both the quality and quantity of sugars a food contains.[1]

3. **Fats** are the major source of stored energy in the body, in humans as well as in other mammals and simpler organisms. Modified fat molecules also play other key roles in the cells that make up the body, such as a central role in generating the membrane that separates all cell content from the blood, and in generating hormones, including steroids. Fats are mostly ingested in the form of triglycerides, which are composed of three chains of carbon and hydrogen molecules (fatty acids) bound together by a molecule of glycerol. After digestion, they are broken down in the intestine by bile salts, released from the gallbladder, and by lipase enzymes released from the pancreas and other organs so they can be absorbed into the blood. Fats can be saturated (when the maximum number of hydrogen atoms are bound to each carbon) or unsaturated (when fewer than the maximum number of hydrogen atoms are bound to each carbon). The unsaturated fats can be divided into monounsaturated fats (such as the oleic acid contained in olive oil) or polyunsaturated fats (such as those contained in salmon and corn oil). The polyunsaturated fats omega-3 and omega-6 are called "essential fatty acids" because the human body cannot generate them, but they are essential for the normal function of cells and organs.

In addition to these three major macronutrients, micronutrients are an essential component of nutrition. Micronutrients, such as vitamins and minerals, account for much of the $37 billion US supplement industry. Yet studies by nutrition expert Dr. Bruce Ames and others show that between 50 and 90 percent of US adults do not get enough vitamin D, E, magnesium, vitamin A, calcium, potassium, or vitamin K. At the same time, several recent articles indicate that dietary supplements containing excess vitamins and minerals are ineffective in preventing major diseases and delaying mortality.[2] One possible exception: a large, randomized, controlled trial reported a minor reduction in cancer and cataracts in people taking daily multivitamins.[3]

Though supplementation with high levels of vitamins and minerals may not protect against aging or diseases, we know they are important for many essential functions of the human body. For example, vitamin D, zinc, and iron are important for normal immune function. Calcium and vitamin D are essential in maintaining normal bone-mineral density.

A diet rich in vegetables, fish, nuts, and whole grains is the ideal way to get the essential nutrients, but even such diets can be deficient in vitamin D and, for vegans and the elderly, vitamin B12. Most people throughout the world who are consuming what is thought of as a high-nourishment diet have similar deficiencies. Because some studies have indicated that high doses of certain vitamins can be toxic, the ideal recommendation, based on the opinion of both supporters and opponents of supplement use, is to take a multivitamin, made by a reputable company, that contains at least vitamin D, E, magnesium, vitamin A, calcium, potassium, or vitamin K, every two to three days.

As I explained in chapter 3, looking for common denominators in support of a given supplement's benefit will ensure that you don't adopt a dietary practice that may later be proved unhealthy. It's possible that in the future, some vitamins or supplements will turn out to have benefits for some aspects of longevity and health, while others may be detrimental. By reducing the supplementation frequency to relatively low doses and two or three times per week, we minimize the chance of a toxic effect while still avoiding malnourishment due to a lack of a particular vitamin or mineral.

Treat Aging: One Hundred at Fifty? Or Fifty at One Hundred?

Nutrition is clearly the most important factor you can take control of to affect how long you live, whether you will be diagnosed with certain major diseases, and whether you will be active and strong or sedentary and frail in old age.

A recent paper examined nearly a thousand men and women who were thirty-eight years old.[4] It found that, in terms of their biological condition, some seemed no older than thirty while others appeared closer to sixty. Furthermore, all those who were biologically older than their true age would continue to age quickly in later years. My students are surprised when I say some centenarians are healthier—and in some ways, younger—than people who are fifty. Clearly this is limited to very few people and certain organs or systems, but it underlines the relative value of knowing someone's chronological age. Maybe one day we will determine how old someone is based not on the year he or she was born, but on his or her biological age, which we are starting to be able to accurately measure.

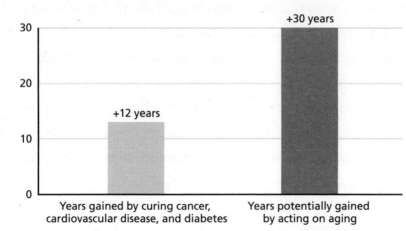

4.1. *Comparison of the potential extension of longevity obtained treating cancer, cardiovascular diseases, and diabetes and delaying aging (with diet, etc.)*

In the remainder of this chapter, I take advantage of the Five Pillars of Longevity to postpone aging and prevent disease by awakening the body's dormant ability to heal, protect, regenerate, and rejuvenate itself.

"I would rather die young than have to eat like that."

When I talk about the Longevity Diet, someone usually makes some variation of the following comment: "I would rather die young than have to eat like that."

It reminds me of the joke about the man who asks his doctor how he can live longer. The doctor recommends he eat very little, give up alcohol, and stop having sex.

"Are you sure it will work?" the man asks.

"I don't really know," the doctor replies, "but no matter how long you live, it will seem an eternity!"

Fortunately, the Longevity Diet isn't *that* restrictive. It allows you to enjoy coffee and alcohol—and puts no limit on sex. Contrary to what you might expect, it often requires that you eat more, not less. As I will describe in detail in chapter 8, a plate of pasta and cheese can weigh just 12 ounces and be very unhealthy, full of bad-quality calories. Or it can weigh more than double that amount, about 1.5 pounds, and be very healthy, full of high-quality calories—provided you cut down the pasta and cheese to modest portions and add plenty of vegetables and legumes and a generous splash of olive oil.

With food, as with most things, people assume anything they want and more of it will make them happier, but that's an illusion. In one of the best TED talks I've seen, Harvard professor Daniel Gilbert compares the happiness of two groups of people: one group had won the lottery; the other was made up of people who had become paraplegic. A year after the life-changing events occurred, both groups were equally happy. In the same way, one's happiness is largely independent of diet. Adopting a diet that promotes a long, healthy lifespan, contrary to what the doctor in the joke says, doesn't make life an unbearable eternity. In fact, I argue that healthier diets can be superior in taste, since vegetables, legumes, nuts, olive oil, and other plant-based foods provide a much wider variety of ingredients and flavors, compared with unhealthy food rich in saturated fats and sugars that obscure natural flavor. I think of the diet high in saturated fat, red meat, fried food, and cheese as equivalent to the sugary drinks most of us consumed when we were children. Eventually, we grew up and started enjoying red wine instead, yet many of us never abandoned the unhealthy food. But it's never too late.

Calorie Restriction: Mice, Monkeys, and Humans

In chapter 2, I described how mice with defects in the growth hormone receptor gene can live up to 50 percent longer than those in the control group, and half of them will not develop detectable diseases. I also described how Ecuadorians with defects in the same gene rarely develop diabetes or cancer and appear to have reduced incidence of other diseases. High protein intake, as I explained, causes the activation of the growth hormone receptor, which in turn increases the levels of insulin and insulin-like growth factor 1 (IGF-1), whose altered concentrations are associated with diabetes and cancer, respectively. Proteins and certain amino acids derived from them, including leucine, can activate TOR-S6K, a set of genes that accelerate aging. Another gene that appears to play a key role in aging is PKA, which we have shown in both simple organisms and mice to be activated by sugars. Mice with reduced PKA activity live longer and are protected against age-related disease.[5]

By reducing calorie intake, particularly reducing calories from proteins and sugars, you can decrease the activities of the growth hormone receptor, and thus of the TOR-S6K and PKA genes known to accelerate aging. These findings represent the "basic/juventology research" pillar, necessary to establish how nutrients act on the aging process.

As a consequence of not recognizing the connection between

proteins and sugars and aging, we have seen the rise over the past thirty years of high-sugar and high-protein diets that have been erroneously labeled "healthy." We are starting to accept that a high-sugar diet is unhealthy. Unfortunately, many are turning to proteins, and in some cases to bad fats, as replacements for sugar. Instead, they should be turning to healthier complex carbohydrates and good fats, as I will explain later in this chapter.

Which diets improve longevity? We have known for nearly one hundred years that when mice are fed about 30 to 40 percent fewer calories, they live longer and develop half the tumors and other diseases when compared to the groups of mice receiving a normal-calorie diet. (An equivalent reduction in a human diet would leave a six-foot-tall man weighing about 130 pounds.) However, since that discovery was made, it's also become clear through multiple further studies of mice and monkeys that chronic caloric restriction can also take a toll. As I mentioned, when I saw my first PhD adviser Roy Walford and the other seven calorie-restricted individuals upon their exit from Biosphere 2 in Arizona, they looked terrible; and as it turns out, those nearly two years of calorie restriction may have cut Walford's life short. He died twelve years later of complications from Lou Gehrig's disease, which many speculate may have been linked to a combination of stress, calorie restriction, and advanced age.

So, on the one hand we know that chronic caloric restriction can have profoundly beneficial effects on risk factors for many diseases. On the other hand, we know that chronic and extreme diets—diets that reduce calories by 20 percent or more and are maintained for long periods or permanently—can negatively affect necessary processes, including wound healing, immune response, and cold-temperature tolerance. Put simply, besides making a person extremely thin, the detrimental effects of chronic calorie restriction appear to minimize its benefits by causing a major increase in other types of diseases and conditions that are less well understood. The focus of the rest of this book is on how to obtain the remarkable beneficial effects of calorie restriction without the negative ones.

The Longevity Diet

What follows is the optimal diet for minimizing disease and maximizing a healthy lifespan based on the Five Pillars.

- **Follow a pescetarian diet.** Aim for a diet that is close to 100 percent plant- and fish-based, limiting fish consumption to two or three portions a week and avoiding fish with high mercury content (tuna, swordfish, mackerel, halibut). If you are past age sixty-five and start to lose muscle mass, strength, and weight, introduce more fish into the diet, along with other animal-based foods commonly consumed by populations with record longevity, like eggs and certain cheeses (preferably feta or pecorino) and yogurt made from goat's milk, all of which are commonly consumed in high-longevity areas.

- **Consume low but sufficient proteins.** Consume 0.31 to 0.36 grams of protein per pound of body weight per day. If you weigh 130 pounds, that comes to about 40 to 47 grams of protein per day, of which 30 grams should be consumed in a single meal to maximize muscle synthesis. If you weigh 200 to 220 pounds and have 35 percent body fat or higher, 60 to 70 grams of protein per day is sufficient, since fat cells require lower levels of protein than muscles. Since this minimum requirement can change from person to person, it is preferable to occasionally consult a dietitian, to make sure that a healthy, lean body mass is maintained. Protein intake should be increased slightly after age sixty-five in individuals who are losing weight and muscle. For most people, a 10 to 20 percent increase (5 to 10 grams more per day) is sufficient. Finally, the diet should be free of animal proteins (red meat, white meat, cheese) with the exception of proteins from fish, but relatively high in vegetable proteins (legumes, nuts, etc.) to minimize the former's negative effects on diseases and maximize the latter's nourishing effects.

■ **Minimize bad fats and sugars, and maximize good fats and complex carbs.** Part of the confusion and constantly changing recommendations around diet stem from the oversimplification of food components and their categorization into fats, carbs, or proteins. Every day we hear about "low carb versus high carb" or "low fat versus high fat." It shouldn't be a question of either/or, but of which type and how much of each. In fact, your diet should be rich in good unsaturated fats, such as those found in olive oil, salmon, almonds, and walnuts, but as low as possible in saturated, hydrogenated, and trans fats. Likewise, the diet should be rich in complex carbohydrates, such as those provided by whole bread, legumes, and vegetables, but low in sugars and limited in pasta, rice, bread, fruit, and fruit juices, which are easily converted into sugars by the time they reach the intestine.

■ **Be nourished.** You can think of the human body as an army of cells always at war. The enemy includes oxygen and other molecules that damage DNA and cells; bacteria; and viruses, which are constantly trying to defeat the immune system. Like an army in need of rations, ammunition, and equipment, the body needs proteins, essential fatty acids (omega-3, omega-6), minerals, vitamins, and, yes, sufficient levels of sugar to fight the many battles raging inside and outside cells. When your intake of certain nutrients becomes too low, the body's repair, replacement, and defense systems slow down or stop, allowing the damage to accumulate or fungi, bacteria, and viruses to proliferate. (The appendixes include a list of foods rich in each of the important nutrients, as well as sample weekly diets that meet established nutritional targets.) As extra insurance, take a multivitamin and mineral pill, plus an omega-3 fish oil soft gel every two or three days. Purchase these products only from reputable companies, where quality control ensures appropriate supplement content and stability.

■ **Eat a variety of foods from your ancestry.** To take in all the required nutrients, you need to eat a wide variety of foods, and it's best to choose from foods that were common on your parents', grandparents', and great-grandparents' table. This does not mean you should eat like your grandparents, but that within the guidelines of this book, you should pick foods your grandparents ate. The human body is the result of billions of years of evolution, and even the last one thousand years have helped filter out people not fit for a particular environment, or foods not appropriate for a particular genotype (the collection of all genes in a person). For example, in many northern European countries where milk was commonly consumed, intolerance to lactose (the sugar contained in milk) is relatively rare, whereas lactose intolerance is very common in southern European and Asian countries, where milk was not historically part of the traditional diet of adults. If a person of Japanese ancestry living in the United States suddenly decides to start drinking milk, which was probably rarely served at her grandparents' table, she will likely start getting sick. Whether it's lactose or kale, quinoa or turmeric (curcumin), you have to ask whether these were foods common at the table when you, your parents, or your grandparents were growing up. If not, it's best to avoid them or consume them only occasionally. The potential problems are intolerances (for example, an inability to break down the lactose sugar in milk) or autoimmunities, such as the reaction to gluten-rich foods like bread and pasta observed in people with celiac disease. Although clear links have not been proved yet, it is possible that consumption of the wrong foods based on ancestry could be associated with many autoimmune disorders, including Crohn's disease, colitis, and type 1 diabetes.

■ **Eat twice a day plus a snack.** Unless your waist circumference and body weight are in the normal or low range, it is best to eat breakfast and one major meal plus a nourishing low-calorie, low-sugar snack daily. If your weight or muscle mass is too low or if it's dropping against your will, then eat three meals a day plus a snack. One of the major mistakes of guidelines on nutrition is blurring the line between what theoretically could work and what actually does work. We often hear that we should eat small meals five to six times a day. Aside from a lack of evidence supporting the benefit of such a regimen in terms of a long and healthy lifespan, it is extremely difficult for most people to regulate food intake when they are told to eat so often. Even if the meals contain 305 calories each, instead of the recommended 300 calories, that extra 30 calories a day, or more than 900 calories a month, means nearly 3 pounds of extra fat every year. Not surprisingly, over the past twenty years—the period when the six-meal diet was popular—America reached a record 70 percent portion of overweight and obese people. If you eat only two and a half meals a day, with only one major meal, it becomes much harder to overeat, particularly on a mostly plant-based diet. It would take large portions of fish, beans, and vegetables to get to the calorie level that would cause obesity. The high nourishment of the food, plus the volume of the meal, signals to your stomach and brain that you have had enough food.

- In the elderly, this one major meal system may have to be broken down into two smaller meals to avoid digestion problems. Older people and adults prone to weight loss should stick to eating three meals a day plus one snack. For people trying to lose weight or those who tend to be heavy, the best nutritional advice is to eat breakfast daily; have lunch or dinner, but not both; and substitute for the missed meal one snack containing fewer than 100 calories and no more than 3 to 5 grams of sugar. (Do not skip breakfast, as this has been associated with increased risk for age-related diseases in multiple studies.) Which meal you skip depends on your lifestyle. The advantage to skipping lunch is more free time and more energy. On the other hand, there is the possible disadvantage of restless sleep from having consumed a large dinner, particularly for those who suffer from acid reflux. The disadvantage to skipping dinner is that it eliminates the most social meal of the day.

- **Observe time-restricted eating.** Another common practice adopted by many centenarian groups is time-restricted eating, or confining all meals and snacks to within eleven to twelve hours or less a day. The efficiency of this method has been demonstrated in both animal and human studies.[6] Typically you would eat breakfast after 8 a.m. and finish dinner before 8 p.m. A shorter eating window (of ten hours or less) can be even more effective for weight loss, but it is much harder to maintain and may increase the risk of side effects, such as developing gallstones and possibly increasing the risk of cardiovascular disease. You should also not eat within three to four hours of going to sleep.

- **Practice periodic prolonged fasting:** People under age sixty-five who are neither frail nor malnourished and are free of major diseases should undergo two periods of five days a year in which they consume a relatively high-calorie fasting-mimicking diet, or FMD. Most religious groups—including Muslims, Christians, Jews, and Buddhists—have practiced some form of fast, though some of these practices have been modified or abandoned over time. Muslims practice fasting during the month of Ramadan, but in modern times the daytime fast is often accompanied by overeating at night. During Lent, Christians used to undergo a month of severe calorie restriction ending in a week of fasting, but this practice, too, has largely been abandoned today. In chapter 6, I discuss the remarkable effects of five-day cycles of a fasting-mimicking diet on disease risk factors and the optimization of healthy longevity.

- **Follow the eight points above in such a way that you reach and maintain a healthy weight and abdominal circumference.** In a longitudinal study of 359,000 European adults followed over ten years, high waist circumference and abdominal fat were associated with increased diabetes, hypertension, high cholesterol, and heart disease. Having a waist circumference of more than 40 inches in men and 35 inches in women doubled the risk of premature death, compared with having a waist circumference of less than 33 inches in men and 27 inches in women. Following the eight points above will allow you to reach and maintain low visceral fat, and a healthy weight and abdominal circumference.

For most people, the Longevity Diet can be adopted simply by replacing a limited number of items with foods that are just as enjoyable, if not more so. Virtually all diets fail because they are too extreme to maintain in the long run. They also fail because they require major changes to your habits and lifestyle. For example, many new diets require low carbohydrate intake, but carbohydrates are the food people around the world enjoy the most—

whether it's potatoes for northern Europeans, pasta for Italians and Americans, or rice for Asians. Thus, very low-carbohydrate diets, besides being associated with increased mortality and reduced lifespan, are not sustainable in the long run for most people. Because the Longevity Diet is closer to diets generally adopted by Americans, Europeans, and Asians, it can be embraced by people all over the world.

In the following sections I explain how the above dietary recommendations are rooted in the Five Pillars of Longevity, since this is the key to understanding their effectiveness. I discuss studies of the laboratories I direct, as well as those of other laboratories and clinics.

Pillar 1: Basic/Juventology Research

It is difficult to perform studies on specific human diets in mice and other simple organisms. However, basic research yields a fundamental understanding of the connection between food components, aging, and disease. For example, we know that proteins (amino acids) consistently accelerate aging in most organisms, including yeast, flies, and mice. We also know that IGF-1 and TOR-S6K, both of which are increased or activated by protein intake, are central promoters of aging and age-related diseases in mice.[7] In a recent study testing many combinations of food components, mice given a low-protein, high-carbohydrate diet lived the longest but also displayed improved health. Mice on a high-protein, low-carbohydrate diet lived the shortest and had the worst health, despite the effect of the diet on weight loss (see fig. 4.2).[8]

In our recent study, we showed that simply by lowering protein intake in mice, we can reduce the incidence of melanoma and breast cancer.[9] Even after tumors were established, their rate of growth slowed in the presence of reduced protein intake. Data from studies in mice and simple organisms also support the role of time-restricted feeding and periodic prolonged fasting in life-span extension and reductions in age-related disease.[10] Recently we also showed that high sugar levels make heart cells and mice more sensitive to damage and death during chemotherapy, confirming our hypothesis that sugar makes cells more vulnerable to damage.[11] Thus basic/juventology research supports the pro-aging role of proteins and sugars.

Pillar 2: Epidemiology

Most large-population studies show an association between longevity and disease prevention, and a diet that is low in protein; largely plant- and fish-based; and rich in complex carbohydrates, olive oil, and nuts. For example, our epidemiological study of six thousand Americans suggested that consuming a high-protein diet is associated with increased levels of the pro-aging growth factor IGF-1 (see fig. 4.3), a 75 percent increased risk of overall mortality, and a three- to fourfold increased risk in cancer mortality compared with consuming the low-protein and plant-based diet recommended here (see fig. 4.4).[12] Contrary to the findings of T. Colin Campbell in The China Study, which advocates consuming low levels of plant-based proteins throughout life, the beneficial effect of a low-protein diet seems to apply only before age sixty-five (fig. 4.3). A Harvard study of nearly 130,000 doctors and nurses also indicates that a low-carb diet high in animal fat and protein is associated with increases in overall cancer and cardiovascular disease mortality, a finding that is in agreement with our research.[13] In line with our previous protein study, a follow-up study of the same group followed by Harvard University, in which I acted as a co-author, showed that consumption of high levels of animal but not plant-based proteins was associated with increased mortality from cardiovascular disease.[14] A similar study of forty thousand men suggests that a low-carb, high-animal-protein diet is associated with a twofold increase in diabetes, a finding also consistent with our discovery in the six-thousand-person protein study.[15] A number of other epidemiological studies consistently associate high IGF-1 levels in the bloodstream with an increase of twofold or more in the incidence of breast, prostate, and other cancer types.[16] Because we know that protein consumption is the key regulator of IGF-1 levels and that animal-protein intake is usually associated with intake of saturated animal fats, these studies bolster the case for a link between cancer, diabetes, and high protein and saturated fat intake.

Epidemiological studies also support the key role of nourishment in disease prevention, since populations with deficiencies in certain vitamins have been shown to have an increased incidence for a variety of diseases. For example, vitamin D deficiency has been associated with an increased risk for diabetes and autoimmune and cardiovascular diseases.[17]

Pillar 3: Clinical Studies

As I've indicated, the gold standard for demonstrating the effect of a food component or diet on longevity and diseases is direct

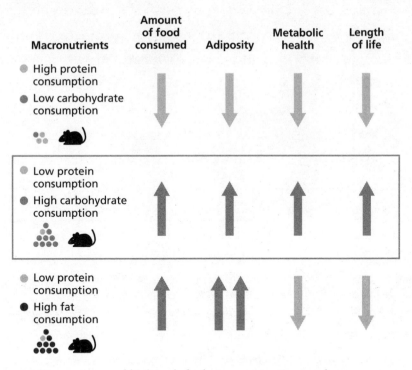

Macronutrients	Amount of food consumed	Adiposity	Metabolic health	Length of life
High protein consumption / Low carbohydrate consumption	↓	↓	↓	↓
Low protein consumption / High carbohydrate consumption	↑	↑	↑	↑
Low protein consumption / High fat consumption	↑	↑↑	↓	↓

4.2. *Low protein and high carbohydrate consumption produces maximum longevity and health in mice.*

testing in a randomized, controlled clinical trial. Subjects are randomly assigned to either a group consuming a control diet (not believed to have an effect on health) or an experimental diet (expected to have a health benefit). A large randomized study to test a longevity diet against a standard diet has not been performed, but we are currently starting several trials aimed at achieving this goal. However, several existing studies do support the recommendations given above. For example, we have shown that even periodic use of a low-protein, plant-based diet can reduce many markers or risk factors for aging and diseases in subjects ages twenty to seventy. (See chapter 6 on fasting and fasting-mimicking diets.) A research group in Spain has randomized people at risk

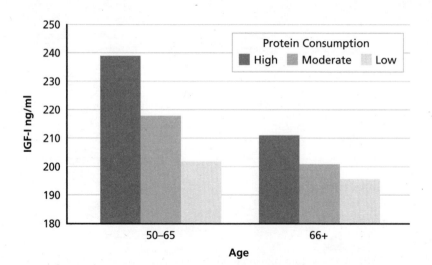

4.3. High levels of IGF-1 (growth factor pro-aging and cancer) are seen only in people with high consumption of protein before age sixty-five.

for cardiovascular diseases to either a "healthy low-fat diet" or a diet rich in olive oil or nuts. A Mediterranean diet with high levels of olive oil or 30 grams a day of nuts (walnuts, hazelnuts, almonds) was associated with reduced cardiovascular events and mortality.[18] The protective role of nuts is also supported by an analysis of many studies investigating their effect on the prevention of multiple diseases.[19] Another set of clinical trials clearly demonstrates that protein intake is associated with high levels of IGF-1, thus supporting the link between proteins, IGF-1, aging, and cancer.

Although it was not a randomized clinical trial, Satchidananda Panda and his colleagues at the Salk Institute studied how the total number of hours that food is consumed daily and when that food is eaten are associated with sleep patterns and risk factors for diseases. They determined that people who consumed food over a

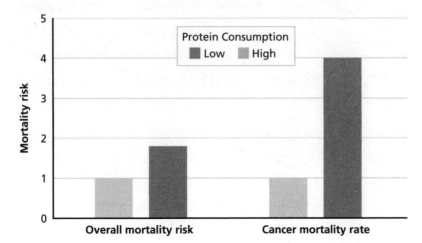

4.4. *High consumption of protein before age sixty-five is sssociated with a 75 percent increase in risk of death and a fourfold increase in risk of death from dancer.*

period of twelve hours or more benefited from reducing the consumption timespan to twelve hours or less.[20] In support of a diet high in complex carbohydrates and good fats being the best even for weight management, when a diet very low in carbohydrates (less than 10 percent of calories) and high in protein (more than 20 percent of calories) and fats was compared with a moderate carbohydrate regimen similar to the Okinawan diet, fat loss was similar in both cases.[21] However, the low-carbohydrate diet caused a much higher loss of water and proteins, indicating that the seemingly large effect of very low-carb diets on weight loss actually represents loss of water and muscle in addition to fat.

Pillar 4: Centenarian Studies

Areas of the world known to have the highest prevalence of centenarians—Okinawa, Japan; Loma Linda, California; small towns in Calabria and Sardinia, Italy; and in Costa Rica and Greece—all share diets that are (1) mostly plant-based with lots of nuts and some fish; (2) low in proteins, sugars, and saturated/trans fats; and (3) high in complex carbohydrates coming from beans and other plant-based foods. Most of these centenarians ate only two or three times a day, ate light meals in the evening, and were in many cases done eating before dark. They also consumed a limited variety of foods—ones typical of their homelands. In some cases they did modify their diet. For example, Okinawans used to get most of their calories from sweet purple potatoes, but today that is far less common.

OKINAWA

Craig Wilcox and his colleagues have compared the dietary habits of typical older people from Okinawa with those of older citizens living in the United States.

As we can see, American seniors ate ten times more meat, poultry, and eggs and three times more fruit, but far less fish, half the vegetables, and one third of the grains that the Okinawans did.

Okinawans	Americans
3% meat/poultry/eggs	29% meat/poultry/eggs
2% dairy/seaweed	23% dairy/seaweed
34% vegetables	16% vegetables
6% fruits	20% fruits
12% soy and similar foods	<1% soy and similar foods
32% grains	11% grains
11% omega-3-rich foods (fish, etc.)	< 1 % fish

4.5. *Dietary habits of Okinawans versus Americans. Willcox, BJ. et al. "Caloric Restriction, the Traditional Okinawan Diet, and Healthy Aging,"* Annals of the New York Academy of Science, *2007.*

Life expectancy (world rank)	Location	Life expectancy	Breast cancer*	Ovarian cancer*	Prostate cancer*	Colon cancer*	Total cancer deaths (% increase versus Okinawa)
1	Okinawa	81.2	6	3	4	8	21 (0)
2	Japan	79.9	11	3	8	16	38 (80%)
4	Sweden	79	34	10	52	19	115 (547%)
8	Italy	78.3	37	4	23	17	81 (368%)
10	Greece	78.1	29	3	20	13	65 (309%)
18	USA	76.8	33	7	28	19	87 (414%)

* Cancer deaths per 100,000 people

4.6. *Risk of hormone-associated cancers (1990s, taken from Okinawa Program). Willcox BJ, et al.* The Okinawa Program, *Harmony, 2002.*

In figure 4.7, we see that far fewer Okinawans have cancer or cardiovascular disease than do Americans or even other people in Japan.

In terms of brain aging and disease, Wilcox and his colleagues report a 30 to 50 percent reduction in the prevalence of dementia in Okinawans of different ages compared with that in people of the same age in the United States.

Other than diet, what makes Okinawans so long-lived? Wilcox and his colleagues believe that physical activity is a key factor for their longevity and health. These activities range from gardening to martial arts to dancing. I observed similar high exercise behavior in elderly individuals when I visited three other zones with high longevity: Loma Linda, California, Sardinia and Calabria, both in Italy. I go into more detail on the connection between exercise and healthy longevity in chapter 5.

Wilcox and his colleagues also report that Okinawans are very

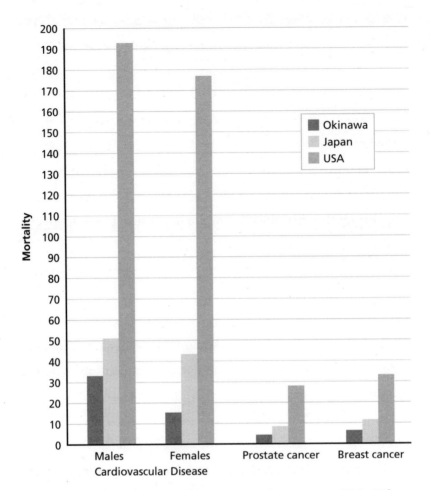

4.7. *Mortality from diseases: Okinawa versus Japan versus USA. Wilcox BJ et al. "Caloric Restriction, the Traditional Okinawan Diet, and Healthy Aging,"* Annals of the New York Academy of Science, 2007.

spiritual, and rely both on doctors and shamans. The effect of spirituality on longevity is less clear than that of diet, but it is often found to be associated with long-lived populations. Many scientific studies suggest that spirituality can be effective in both preventing and treating some diseases and medical conditions. Having interviewed centenarians all over the world, I think the common denominator is not spirituality per se, but a sense of purpose, a will to live. A distinguished colleague once told me his theory: "What many of the longest-lived people in the world have in common," he said, "is that they are tough. They are fighters, and they will go on even when their own children have died." As did Jeanne Calment of France, who reached the record age of 122, outliving both her daughter and grandson by several decades. Calment quit smoking at 117, not for health reasons, but because she became too blind to light up by herself and refused to ask for help. Famously witty, she is known to have said, "I've only got one wrinkle, and I'm sitting on it."

Although it will be difficult to ever quantify this, my conclusion is that some centenarians find their strength in God, some in their families, but many find it in the joy of living—in tasting an egg after going through years of war and famine when they could only dream of eggs, or simply drinking a glass of wine. Which brings me to Italy, and two of my favorite people in the world.

SALVATORE CARUSO AND MOLOCHIO, ITALY

Although my grandparents died years ago, and even my mother and father rarely go back, I have always remembered the many summers I spent in Molochio, and even after settling down in Los Angeles I continued to visit. I thought this little village, lost in the Aspromonte mountains, was worth a stop on my yearly visit home to Italy, and so were its people—but I never could have imagined that the elderly people of the little town that holds so many fond childhood memories for me would serve as a confirmation of our discoveries about nutrition and longevity in the lab and epidemiological surveys among US populations.

It was around 2006, and my uncle in Molochio, the village of two thousand people where both my parents grew up, told me that Salvatore Caruso had reached one hundred years of age. Big deal, I thought. But I remembered Salvatore, *u ragiuniere* (the accountant), who was well known for the interesting stories he told. He had even written a book chronicling his life.

Year after year, the number of centenarians kept on increasing and by 2010, four villagers had reached the age of one hundred. So I started visiting Salvatore and a few others, and I started asking questions about their lifestyle and diet. In addition to the invaluable information about diet and longevity, a great gift from these centenarians is their ability to recall one hundred years of adventures, wars, and stories of all kinds in seconds, to surprise you and make you laugh. Soon I realized that Molochio had one of the highest concentrations of centenarians in the world.

Salvatore, who also owned land where he tended olive trees, always said his credo was *"No Bacco, no tobacco, no Venere,"* which didn't make him very popular around town, since it means no Bacchus (wine), no smoking, no Venus (women). As with most centenarians, however, the stories they tell can be very different from the facts; as it happens, Salvatore was married with children and liked to drink wine regularly. I did not have to ask much about his diet, since it was the same as my grandfather's: dark bread, olives, olive oil, walnuts, almonds, stockfish, tomatoes, and most of all and almost every day, *pasta e vaianeia*, the pasta dish with lots of vegetables and beans, including green beans in the pod. Variations on this dish still represent the most frequent meals at my own table.

Why did Salvatore, my grandfather, and everyone else in Molochio eat all those beans? Because they were grown locally and were all they could afford. Not surprisingly, hardship played a key role in the historical diet of this region. In one of the documentaries filmed in Molochio, a French television journalist asked one of the other centenarians of Molochio how many times per week she ate meat in her younger years. At first, she didn't understand the question. When her daughter translated in the local dialect, she started to laugh. "Meat, yes, I had meat. My friends and I snuck into a wedding one time and we ate meat." We are so accustomed to thinking about meat consumption in terms of times per week that we did not realize that for some of the Molochio centenarians, the opportunities to eat meat were rare.

A few years later, I was in another magical place I like to visit every year—the mountains of southern Ecuador, where I was studying the villagers with Laron syndrome—I was interviewed

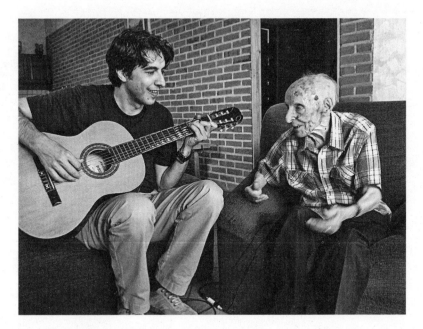

4.8. With Salvatore Caruso

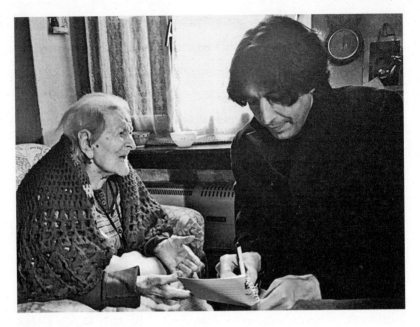

4.9. With Emma Morano

by journalist Stephen Hall, who was writing a cover story on parts of the world with extraordinary longevity for *National Geographic* (May 2013 issue). I told him about my grandfather's village. "If you really want to meet people who make it to very old age without disease, then you must go to my parents' hometown," I told him. Stephen asked a few questions, but probably thought the same thing I did: it sounds a little too convenient. To my surprise, several months later he emailed me from there. "I'm in Molochio," he wrote, "and I just confirmed that there are four centenarians and four 99-year-olds among its 2,000 inhabitants." The Molochio centenarians became the centerpiece of the story.

One key observation, made in collaboration with my colleague Giuseppe Passarino, is that the Molochian centenarians tend to live with their sons' or daughters' families. Because the younger generation has adopted a more modern diet, we speculated that transitioning to a higher-protein diet with more animal-based ingredients—which many of the centenarians did in their eighties and nineties—may contribute to their extreme longevity. In other words, maintaining a high-vegetable, low-protein diet for the first seventy or eighty years of life, and later switching to a diet richer in proteins but also animal-based foods like eggs, chicken, milk, and certain cheeses, may have slowed down aging and optimized the health of the Molochio centenarians. This explanation fits with our discovery that low-protein intake is associated with extended longevity and a major reduction in cancer in people age sixty-five and younger, but not in those above sixty-six.[22] In fact, we know that IGF-1 and other hormones that contribute to aging can reach very low levels after age eighty. This may make a strict low-protein diet less beneficial against cancer and diabetes in later life, as well as a risk factor for frailty and defects in the immune system and wound healing. Again, this problem does not require complex changes and is solved by maintaining the Longevity Diet until age sixty-five or seventy, then gradually increasing one's level of protein and general nourishment by 10 to 20 percent to maintain a healthy weight and muscle strength.

EMMA MORANO, VERBANIA, ITALY

Another one of my favorite people was Emma Morano, of Verbania, Italy. Emma died in 2017 at age 117. Records show that Emma is the oldest Italian ever to have lived, and up until her death she held the title of the oldest living person in the world. A reporter from *The New York Times* asked me why Emma, who ate three eggs a day and consumed plenty of meat, was one of the longest-lived women in human history. My response, as quoted in the article: "If you take 100 centenarians, you get 100 different elixirs of longevity."[23]

It turns out that although she ate eggs and meat in her old age, Emma's diet was probably much more plant-based, with lots of rice and minestrone, for many decades of her life. More important, Emma probably had the right genes, which can increase by manyfold the chance that someone will live to 100. Her mother had died at 94, her sister at 102, two other sisters had reached 98, and her brother passed away at 90.

Research shows that the sons of centenarians have an overall 50 percent reduction of disease onset for hypertension, stroke and seizure, cardiac disease, and diabetes. According to these data, having just one parent who lives past the age of 87 reduces your chances of getting cancer by 24 percent.[24] This is analogous to something we saw among the Laron people of Ecuador: the rare individuals who maintain a very unhealthy diet become overweight or obese but still live a long and healthy life. Furthermore, Emma was under the care of an excellent physician, Dr. Carlo Bava, whose medical decisions for the past thirty years undoubtedly contributed to her record longevity.

Scientists are trying to test and produce drugs capable of causing the same effects as the genetic mutations that extend the healthy lifespan, but those won't be available for many years. For now, the food we eat is the most potent intervention available for disease prevention and treatment.

Emma remembered a lot, but the things she talked about most were the death of her son—at only seven months of age—and how she packed her bags and left her ex-husband after he abused her. That had happened in her late thirties, nearly eighty years in the past by the time she was telling me her stories. I was also impressed by how protective she was of her photo album, not letting me touch it and swatting my hand away whenever I got too close. She was letting me know that she would be needing it for a long time to come.

Her zest for life was evident in other ways too. When we visited Emma in 2015, a researcher from my group proposed to bring a scarf as a present. But I thought it might be better to bring something Emma could enjoy more. So we brought her a cake made of fruit. When I gave Emma the cake, she was tired and absentminded, so she didn't say anything about the cake. Her reaction made me think she didn't like it and maybe it would have been better to bring her a scarf. As we exchanged greetings, one of her nieces said: "Don't worry, Aunt. I'll put the cake right there, next to you, close to the pillow." After just five minutes, Emma was eating the cake enthusiastically. Ten minutes later, the cake was gone. Emma had devoured it in a very organized way, feeding herself without dropping a crumb. She also had a bowl of soup and some eggs.

SARDINIA: THE ISLAND OF LONGEVITY

Although I'm only now beginning to follow the centenarians of the Nuoro region of Sardinia, Italy, researchers Gianni Pes, Michel Poulain, and Luca Deiana, as well as author Dan Buettner, have made this region world famous. Certain villages in Sardinia's blue zone have had the number of centenarians reach levels among the highest observed anywhere in the world and possibly even higher than those of Molochio.

Nowadays many regions (Russia and South America, in particular) claim to have high longevity zones. But the stories about longevity coming out of these areas are often invented by inhabitants who want to lure journalists and tourists. Sardinia, on the other hand, is an area of record longevity validated by demographers. The Sardinians eat a diet that is probably familiar to you by now: mostly plant-based, with beans, whole-grain breads, and lots of vegetables. Because of high local production, they also consume pecorino, the high omega-3 cheese made from ewe's milk.

LOMA LINDA: CALIFORNIA'S LAND OF LONGEVITY

An hour's drive from Los Angeles is a Seventh-day Adventist church that has been under close scrutiny by Dr. Gary Fraser and others of Loma Linda University. When researchers compared the longevity of Californians belonging to this church with the longevity of all Californians, they found that the Adventist men—who are vegetarians—lived nearly ten years longer than the average California man. Adventist women lived on average six years longer than California women in general.[25] Again, not surprisingly, among the very long-lived vegetarian California Adventists, those who consumed nuts at least five times a week, two or more servings of vegetables per day, and three or more servings of legumes per week lived the longest and had reduced incidence of disease. Other common characteristics of California Adventists, besides vegetarianism, are eating light dinners early, exercising often, and maintaining a healthy weight and abdominal circumference. Even in Southern California, the center for fad diets, members of the longest-lived community consume lots of vegetables, legumes, walnuts, and almonds, which they spread across two or three daily meals served within twelve hours.

Pillar 5: Studies of Complex Systems

This is clearly the most abstract of the pillars, but it can play an important supporting role in reaching solid conclusions. For example, we can better understand the effect of age on the requirement for higher protein and food intake in elderly and frail Americans, and in centenarians, by considering how poorly maintained cars may lose fuel efficiency as they get older. Another way to use complex systems like cars or planes to understand human aging is by comparing the complicated nourishment of the human body to not only gasoline (the source of energy) but also brake fluid, radiator coolant, and motor oil. For example, the radiator is not involved in running the car, but its ability to cool the engine makes it essential for the car's longevity.

In either the human body or a car, low fluid level—even of fluids needed for a relatively minor subsystem, such as the radiator—can accelerate aging and cause the whole system to break down. Undernourishment in humans is like low levels of motor oils or other fluids in cars. Another comparison: the car—like the human body—needs both high-quality oils and fuel for its brakes and engine to operate properly. If these products are of low quality or the wrong kind—similar to saturated fats in our diet—the engine and other parts of the car can be damaged and deteriorate faster. Eventually the damage will lead to car problems that must be fixed, just as the aging process in humans leads to diseases. These analogies help simplify the complexity of human biochemistry and underline the fundamental link between nutrients, their functions, aging, and disease. As I have already mentioned, whereas the correct levels of proteins, unsaturated fats, and carbohydrates are beneficial, excess levels of proteins, saturated fats, and sugars can accelerate aging and damage the human body. This is not surprising, considering that humans have evolved in an environment where proteins, sugars, and saturated fats were rarely available at high levels for long periods.

The Longevity Diet in Summary

1. Eat mostly vegan, plus a little fish, limiting meals with fish to a maximum of two or three times per week. Choose fish, crustaceans, and mollusks with a high omega-3, omega-6, and vitamin B12 content (salmon, anchovies, sardines, cod, sea bream, trout, clams, shrimp; see appendix B). Pay attention to the quality of the fish, choosing those with low levels of mercury.

2. If you are below the age of sixty-five, keep the intake of protein low (0.31 to 0.36 grams per pound of body weight). That comes to 40 to 47 grams of protein per day for a person weighing 130 pounds, and 60 to 70 grams of protein per day for someone weighing 200 to 220 pounds. Those beyond age sixty-five should slightly increase their protein intake, in-

cluding fish, eggs, white meat, and products derived from goats and sheep, to preserve muscle mass. Consume beans, chickpeas, green peas, and other legumes as your main source of protein.

3. Minimize saturated fats from animal and vegetable sources (meat, cheese) and sugar, and maximize good fats and complex carbs. Eat whole grains and high quantities of vegetables (tomatoes, broccoli, carrots, legumes, etc.) with generous amounts of olive oil (3 tablespoons per day) and nuts (1 ounce per day). See the biweekly diet program in appendix A.

4. Follow a diet with high vitamin and mineral content and complete it with a multivitamin buffer every 3 days.

5. Select ingredients among those discussed in this book that your ancestors would have eaten.

6. Based on your weight, age, and abdominal circumference, decide whether to have two or three meals per day (see chapter 8 for diabetes guidelines). If you are overweight or tend to gain weight easily, consume two meals a day: breakfast and either lunch or dinner, plus two low-sugar (less than 5 grams) snacks with fewer than 100 calories each. If you are already at a normal weight, or if you tend to lose weight easily or are over 65 and of normal weight, eat three meals a day and one low-sugar (less than 3 to 5 grams) snack with fewer than 100 calories.

7. Confine all eating to within a twelve-hour period; for example, start after 8 a.m. and end before 8 p.m. Don't eat anything within three to four hours of bedtime.

8. Until age 65–70, depending on weight and frailty, undergo five days of a fasting-mimicking diet (see chapter 6) every one to six months, based on your goals and, if possible, a dietitian's or medical doctor's advice.

9. Follow points 1 through 8 in such a way that you reach and maintain a healthy weight and abdominal circumference.

Chapter 5

Exercise and Healthy Longevity

A Lesson from Centenarians

In general, those who reach age one hundred in good health have stayed active or very active into old age. There are of course exceptions. If you look at centenarians, or even just within your own extended family, you will likely find someone who beat the odds: eating whatever they wanted, seldom exercising, yet making it to a ripe old age. Nir Barzilai of the Albert Einstein College of Medicine studies Ashkenazi Jewish centenarians in New York, many of whom are completely sedentary, he reports. Their longevity is likely due to genetics. Clearly genes are the most powerful factor in determining lifespan. We know this because we have identified mutations that cause a high degree of protection against age-related diseases in both mice and humans. We also know that a chimpanzee can eat the perfect diet and exercise regularly yet never come close to the average human lifespan. Despite sharing 95 percent of our DNA sequence, chimps rarely live beyond age fifty. There is nothing we can do about our genes. But after making changes in the diet, the second major factor affecting lifespan is physical activity.

In Okinawa, I heard stories of fishermen who never retire, and I watched a woman in her nineties dance with a large bottle on her head, something she did many times a week. When she wasn't dancing, she enjoyed playing traditional Japanese musical instruments. In Calabria, 110-year-old Salvatore Caruso told me how he walked every day to the *oliveto* (olive grove) and how much labor his olive trees required. In Loma Linda, the very long-lived Seventh-day Adventists are famous for their high levels of exercise, including walking fast and going to the gym.[1] When Dan Buettner asked very long-lived Costa Ricans to share the secret to their longevity, they said they enjoyed doing physical work all their lives. When I posed the same question to the shepherds of towns with famously long-lived populations in Sardinia, they told me that every year they left their homes around November so they could walk their sheep to lower elevations and warmer areas, where the animals can find food, and they didn't return until April or May.[2]

What physical activity is best for healthy longevity? The one you enjoy most, but also the one you can easily incorporate into your daily schedule and the one you can keep doing up to your hundredth birthday and beyond. Many Okinawans practice martial arts, especially a dance-inspired version of tai chi. The type of exercise you choose isn't important. What's important is working all your body parts until you breathe rapidly and sweat for five to ten hours a week.

I'm not talking about running weekly marathons. Overworking your body is not a good idea. If you consider the "complex systems" pillar described earlier and think about a car, why is it that no one wants to buy a five-year-old car with one hundred thousand miles on the odometer? Because despite being relatively new, it has been driven too much. You can replace the tires and repaint the chassis, but you cannot change every belt, hose, and valve, and there's a high chance that some overworked component will break down. On the other hand, you don't want to leave your car parked in the garage most of the time, as this will also eventually cause it to break down.

The same holds true for the human body. It's important to exercise, but not to overexercise, because knees, hips, and joints will eventually get damaged—particularly if you continue to exercise when you feel pain. On the bright side, certain exercises and diet can cause tissue to self-repair and regenerate, so the human body has built-in advantages over a car.

Optimizing Exercise for Longevity

The following guidelines are for exercising to maximize health and longevity:

Walk fast for an hour every day. The goal of walking for an hour a day can easily be achieved. For example, pick a coffee shop or restaurant fifteen minutes from your work and make a point of going there twice a day. It can also be achieved on the weekend by walking when you would normally drive. Every year, I take my USC students from Los Angeles to Genoa, Italy, for three weeks. On the first day, we do a walking tour of the city. I then urge them to continue walking everywhere for the duration of the trip. By the end of the course, they are used to walking around the city and realize that they enjoy it and feel better in general.

Ride, run, or swim thirty to forty minutes every other day, plus two hours on the weekend. The best way to achieve this goal is to have both a stationary bike and a road bike. When you can, ride outside; when you can't, use the exercise bike in high gear (use a bike that provides the option of high magnetic resistance, which makes it hard to pedal—as if you were going uphill). After ten minutes, you should be sweating. If you ride on the street, go uphill for at least ten to fifteen minutes. Do this for about forty minutes every other day and for two hours on the weekend.

Bicycling may be healthier than running because it minimizes stress on the joints. However, a long-term study showed that long-distance running among healthy older adults was not associated with osteoarthritis,[3] so an injury caused by long-distance running may be less common than we would expect. In fact, another study that followed 74,752 runners for seven years concluded that running reduced both weight and the risk of osteoarthritis.[4]

Following one pillar of longevity (studies of complex systems), we could conclude that bicycling is preferable to running. But following another pillar (epidemiology), running would appear to be equally good. Its beneficial effects, however, may change over time and may vary in individuals who are injured, have joint damage, and continue to run. Thus, I would recommend a bicycle as a first choice, but running is also fine if the limits described below are followed. Swimming is another excellent form of exercise, although its beneficial effects on longevity have received less scrutiny than those of running.

Use your muscles. Humans evolved as a species that walks, runs, climbs trees and hills, and uses a variety of muscles all the time. Now people use elevators and escalators instead of stairs, drive instead of walk, use dishwashers and washing machines instead of washing dishes and clothes by hand, buy food instead of growing it, and hire people to do even minor repair work around the house instead of fixing things ourselves.

Every muscle of the body needs to be used frequently, because muscles grow and maintain or gain strength only in response to being challenged. Climbing six flights of stairs rapidly can cause leg pain, especially if you haven't done it in a long time. That pain is evidence of minor injury to your muscles. In the presence of sufficient amounts of proteins, muscle injury leads to the activation of "muscle satellite cells" and, eventually, to muscle growth. Muscles can be slightly injured and rebuilt by doing simple every-day tasks that are challenging. Of course, minor injury can turn into major injury if the burden in weight-bearing exercise is too high or if you keep reinjuring already inflamed muscle or cartilage. Muscle training must be balanced to avoid both acute injuries and the slow, chronic damage that comes with ignoring pain and continuing to put stress on an injured joint.

Exercise Length, Strength, and Efficacy

How long and how strenuously should you exercise to optimize healthy longevity? Most studies linking exercise and longevity are sustained by just a single pillar, epidemiology, which is insufficient to reliably conclude a primary role for exercise in longer life. Nonetheless, exercise and longevity studies still provide very valuable information, particularly when hundreds of thousands of subjects are followed.

An Australian study looking for a link between exercise and longevity monitored 204,542 people ages forty-five to seventy-five for eight years. The group reporting more than 150 minutes a week of moderate to vigorous exercise displayed a 47 percent reduction in overall mortality, while the group exercising at moderate to vigorous levels for 300 minutes per week had a 54 percent reduction, so twice as much exercise did not provide much additional benefit.[5] The effect was increased by another 9 percent in those who sometimes exercised vigorously.

Metabolic equivalent tasks (METs) are commonly used to

Light: up to 3 METs	Moderate: 3 to 6 METs	Vigorous: over 6 METs
Slow walking	Fast walking >4 mph	Climbing stairs/hiking
Slow bicycling	Bicycling 10–12 mph	Bicycling >12 mph
Standing, doing light work	Gardening	Playing soccer
Doing office work	Slow jogging	Jogging >6 mph

5.1. *Exercise levels and corresponding activities.*

express the intensity of physical activity. One MET is defined as the energy cost of sitting quietly and is equivalent to a caloric consumption of 1 kilocalorie per kilogram per hour. Moderate exercise involves movement that burns three to six times the calories used when sitting still (3 to 6 METs). Vigorous exercise burns calories at more than six times the resting level (more than 6 METs).

Another very large study, combining data from six studies performed in the United States and Europe, followed 661,137 men and women (with a median age of sixty-two) over fourteen years. During that period, 116,686 participants died. The data showed that even those who exercised less than 150 minutes at moderate intensity or 75 minutes at vigorous intensity per week had a 20 percent reduced risk of mortality compared with those who did not exercise. Mortality was reduced by 31 percent in those who exercised for more than 150 minutes a week at moderate intensity or for more than 75 minutes a week at vigorous intensity. And the risk of dying was reduced by 37 percent in those exercising more than 300 minutes a week at moderate intensity or 150 minutes at high intensity.[6] Again, the difference between exercising for 150 or

300 minutes was minimal. Exercising more than this resulted in very minor additional health benefits, but the study showed a trend for a potentially less beneficial effect among those who exercised ten times the recommended minimum.

Protein Intake and Weight Training

High protein intake is believed by most to be necessary to maintain or increase muscle mass. However, several studies indicate that exceeding a daily protein intake of 0.33 grams per pound of body weight does not increase muscle growth and that consuming 30 grams of protein in a single low-carbohydrate or very low-carbohydrate meal optimizes muscle synthesis.[7] For best results, the 30 grams of protein should be consumed one to two hours after resistance training, such as lifting weights or doing push-ups. In both young and older individuals, the ideal muscle synthesis occurred when the weight being lifted or pushed was 60 to 75 percent of one's maximum capacity.[8]

OPTIMIZING ENERGY IN SUMMARY

1. Walk fast for an hour every day.
2. Take the stairs instead of escalators and elevators.
3. On the weekend, walk everywhere, even faraway places (avoid polluted areas as much as you can).
4. Do moderate exercise for 2½ to 5 hours a week, with some of it in the vigorous range. Most of the beneficial effects appear to be caused by the first 2.5 hours of exercise, making the additional exercise optional.

5. Use weight training or weight-free exercises to strengthen all muscles.

6. To maximize muscle growth, consume at least 30 grams of protein in a single meal one to two hours after a relatively intense weight-training session.

Chapter 6

Fasting-Mimicking Diets, Weight Management, and Healthy Longevity

AS I MENTIONED EARLIER, IN 1992, when I saw my mentor Roy Walford exit Biosphere 2 after nearly two years of a severe calorie-restricted diet, I looked at Roy and the other seven emaciated Biospherians and thought, "There must be a better way to delay aging and prevent disease." Ten years later, as I was searching for ways to protect cancer patients while leaving their cancer cells vulnerable to therapy, I remembered the baker's yeast experiments from my doctoral research at UCLA. Moving yeast cells from a sugar-rich medium into a medium of pure water had protected them from various toxins, and also caused cells to live twice as long. We eventually determined that switching mice from their normal high-calorie diet to water also protected them from damage caused by the same toxins. And since we knew that both humans and monkeys kept on chronic calorie restriction were at risk for side effects—immune system deficiencies, problems with wound healing, extremely low weight, and high levels of stress, to name a few—I wondered: Could the protective effect of short periods of fasting continue after the mice returned to a normal diet? If so, we could design a periodic short-term fast that would be easy to implement. The burden would be minimal, and the timing and frequency would be within the individual's control. By limiting the period of fasting to four to five days no more than once a month we could also minimize the side effects.

It was a great plan in theory, but when we tested water-only fasting in cancer patients, the three-day trial was not exactly a roaring success. Not because the results were bad—they were in fact very promising—but because the patients, who were undergoing chemotherapy at the time, found it difficult to undergo such an extreme fast, and their doctors and nurses were also very resistant to the idea (see chapter 7 for more on cancer prevention and treatment). So we needed to find a different solution.

In our cancer studies with mice, we had determined that four major changes in the blood need to occur to show that the mouse had entered a protected state as a result of fasting: (1) lower levels of the growth factor IGF-1; (2) lower levels of glucose; (3) higher levels of ketone bodies, the by-product of fat breakdown; and (4) higher levels of a growth factor inhibitor (IGFBP1).

To achieve these results (i.e., to mimic fasting), we fine-tuned a diet low in proteins and sugars and rich in healthy fats. We took advantage of many additional nutritechnologies developed in my lab to ensure proper nourishment and maximum therapeutic effects. We called this regimen the fasting-mimicking diet (FMD), and later developed it into the product ProLon.

When we tested the three-day-long ProLon in sixteen-month-old mice (the equivalent of a forty-five-year-old human), the results were remarkable:

- Their 75 percent lifespan (that is, the age at which 75 percent of the mice were still alive) was extended by 18 percent. Their 50 percent lifespan grew by 11 percent.
- The mice ate the same quantities of food per month as the mice on the non-ProLon diet, yet they lost weight, primarily abdominal fat, without loss of muscle mass.
- Age-dependent loss of bone mineral density dropped.
- Tumors were reduced by nearly half, and cancer onset for the great majority of mice on ProLon was pushed back to twenty-six months (equivalent to approximately seventy years for humans) from the onset at twenty months (equivalent to approximately age sixty in humans) in the group on the normal diet. Furthermore, the abnormal lesions in mice on Prolon tended to occur in no more than two organs, indicating that many tumors were probably benign.
- Skin inflammatory disorders were cut in half.
- In the ProLon group, a stem cell–dependent regenerative process rejuvenated the immune system. Regeneration also occurred in the liver, muscle, and brain. Levels of several types of stem cells increased.
- In three different cognitive tests, old mice in the ProLon group performed better at motor coordination (movement), learning, and remembering than the control group.

Consistent with our ProLon research in middle-age mice, we showed in several other mouse studies discussed in the following

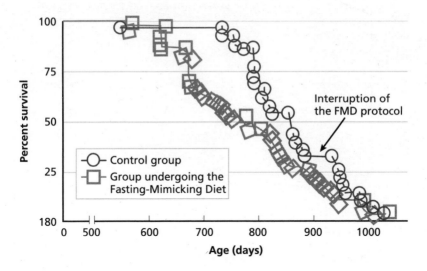

6.1. *Mice receive FMD twice a month from the age of sixteen months.*

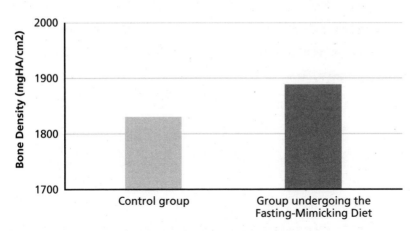

6.2. *Old mice exposed to FMD show less bone density loss (mgHa) when compared with those in the control group.*

chapters that periodic fasting promotes stem cell–dependent regeneration in the immune system, nervous system, and pancreas. The fasting itself destroys many damaged cells, and damageed components inside the cells but it also activates stem cells. Once the mice begin eating again, these stem cells become part of a

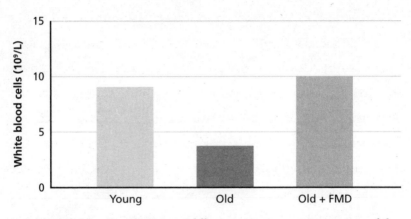

6.3. *Mice that receive FMD in middle age experience rejuvenation of the immune system.*

program to regenerate the organ or system, with the newly regenerated cells bearing characteristics of younger, more functional cells.[1] Additionally, the inside of a variety of cells is partially rebuilt as part of a process called autophagy, also contributing to cellular rejuvenation.

Effects of ProLon in Humans: A Hundred-Subject Clinical Trial

These remarkable results from the mouse studies prompted us to develop an equivalent fasting-mimicking diet for humans. Unlike the one we had developed for cancer patients (see chapter 7), this FMD would have enough calories, vitamins, minerals, and essential nutrients to require minimal medical supervision.

Abstaining from food is a tradition that goes back thousands of years. Early Christians performed the Black Fast during Lent, Muslims fast during Ramadan, and Hindus set aside one day a week for fasting. While little is known about the frequency of fasting in prehistoric times, it's certain that periodic prolonged fasting was common among our Paleolithic and Neolithic ancestors. Religious fasting has been all but abandoned in modern times; among Christians, the Lenten practice of forty days of calorie restriction ending in a week of water-only fasting has almost disappeared, and the traditional Ramadan fasting month, meant to be a period of restriction and self-discipline during the day, nowadays is often accompanied by overeating after sunset. But the mere fact that fasting is historically common to most religions supports the idea that fasting is not a fad diet, but part of our history and evolution. However, religious fasting was not and is not done for health reasons, so it was important to identify a length and type of fasting that is in fact beneficial for health, while minimizing the burden and safety concerns associated with fasting. A label that is now widely used by the media is "Intermittent Fasting." I believe this represents a problematic direction because, like the "Mediterranean Diet" or "eating in moderation" it allows people to improvise and pick and choose periods of fasting that range from 12 hours to weeks, giving the impression that just because they all involve some period of "abstention from food" they are similar or equivalent and all provide health benefits. In fact, they have very different effects. For example, if we consider fasting as the period necessary to switch from a primarily sugar-burning mode to a fat-burning mode, then only periods of abstention from food lasting two or three days or more can be considered fasting. The same length of fasting appears to be necessary to trigger the activation of "regenerative" programs. This does not mean that shorter periods of abstention from food cannot be beneficial, but that we should not use words like "Intermittent Fasting" to include interventions that are very different and have very different effects just like we don't want to place in the same category walking for fifteen minutes and running a marathon.

We have abundant safety data on long-term fasting from such programs as Northern California's TrueNorth Health Center and the Buchinger Wilhelmi clinics in Germany and Spain, where thousands of patients a year undergo fasts of a week or longer supervised by medical staff. Because these fasting regimens are either water-only (TrueNorth) or confined to a few hundred calories per day (Buchinger Wilhelmi), it is important to do this in a specialized clinic and under medical supervision. Some doctors and nutritionists offer outpatient fasting support, but this requires expertise and can be dangerous.

By contrast, the five-day FMD was developed with the following goals:

1. To provide sufficient calories to be safe outside of a clinic
2. To provide a variety of components that most people can enjoy
3. To be 100 percent plant-based, as described in the Longevity Diet in chapter 4
4. To be equally effective as fasting, if not more so

The FMD, as demonstrated in our animal studies, treats aging and promotes healthy longevity using the following processes:

■ Switching all cells to a protected anti-aging mode
■ Promoting autophagy (self-eating of parts of the cell) and replacing damaged cell components with newly generated functional ones

- Killing damaged cells in many organs and systems and replacing them with newly regenerated cells from activated stem cells
- Shifting the body into an abdominal/visceral fat-burning mode, which continues after returning to a normal diet (probably due to epigenetic changes, which are modifications of the DNA and proteins that bind DNA)

Our randomized study of one hundred patients carried out at the USC medical center yielded impressive results. Participants who adopted an FMD for five days a month over a period of three months showed remarkable outcomes in the following areas:

Weight loss	More than 8 pounds in obese subjects, much of that from shedding abdominal fat
Muscle mass	Increased relative to body weight
Glucose	12 mg/dL decrease in subjects with high fasting-glucose (prediabetic) and a return to the normal range for prediabetic subjects; no effect in participants with low fasting-glucose
Blood pressure	6 mmHg decrease in subjects with moderately high blood pressure, but not in subjects with low blood pressure
Cholesterol	20 mg/dL decrease in participants with high cholesterol
IGF-1 (associated with a high cancer risk)	55 ng/mL decrease in participants in the higher-risk range
C-reactive protein (CRP; a risk factor for cardiovascular disease)	1.5 mg/dL decrease and, in most cases, a return to normal levels in participants with elevated CRP
Triglycerides	A 25 mg/dL decrease in participants with high triglycerides

6.4. Reduction in risk factors for diabetes, cancer, and cardiovascular diseases after three cycles of the FMD (one hundred subjects randomized clinical trial)

Three months after the last ProLon FMD cycle, test subjects still benefited from a significant loss of body fat and reductions in waist circumference, glucose levels, IGF-1, and blood pressure, all of which suggests that the use of the FMD every three months may be sufficient to reduce the risk of a number of diseases.

Awakening the Rejuvenation from Within

If a forty-five-year-old couple can have a near-perfect baby, then clearly the adult body holds all the information necessary to generate a new and viable set of cells, organs, and systems without transferring any of the damage present in the original oocyte and sperm cell. But is it possible to trigger the same regenerative process within adult organisms?

Perhaps I'm biased because it was my group that discovered its

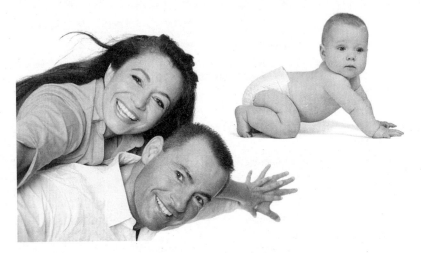

6.5. The sperm cell and egg of a couple in their forties can create a perfect baby.

beneficial effects, but I believe the FMD is probably the best way to start this regenerative and self-healing process, with minimal or potentially no side effects (see my TEDx talk, "Fasting: Awakening the Rejuvenation from Within," on YouTube). The randomized clinical trial results outlined above were achieved in just three months after three cycles of five-day FMD using human subjects. The findings are in keeping with our mouse studies, which showed that FMD acts by breaking down and regenerating the inside of cells (autophagy) and killing off and replacing damaged cells (regeneration). In fact, both in humans and mice, we detected a transient elevation of circulating stem cells in the blood during FMD, which may be responsible for the regeneration and rejuvenation occurring in multiple systems.

By feeding people a very specific diet that tricks the organism into a starvation mode, most organs and systems eliminate unnecessary components (proteins, mitochondria, etc.) but also kill off many cells. As a result, the organism saves energy because it needs to maintain fewer and less active cells. In addition, both cells that are killed and cellular components broken down by

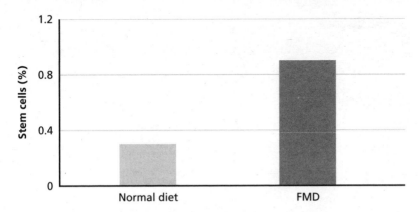

6.6. *Blood stem cells in patients during FMD*

autophagy can provide energy to other cells. A good analogy is to think of the body as an old wood-burning steam locomotive low on wood. To reach the next fueling station, the fireman can start burning the train's oldest and most damaged wooden seats and walls, making the train lighter while generating the steam needed to keep it going. Just as the seats can be rebuilt once the train reaches the fueling station, the streamlined cells, systems, and organs can be rebuilt by activating stem or progenitor cells and activating repair and replacement systems inside the cell to cause regeneration—once the body resumes normal feeding patterns.

FMD Versus Drugs
and Stem Cell–Based Therapies

Many promoters of alternative medicine avoid traditional medicine and even new technologies entirely. Similarly, many doctors and scientists searching for new therapies avoid alternative and natural interventions at all costs. This is a mistake on both sides, and will often mean that a therapy or preventive measure is only partly effective.

In chapter 7, I show how the combination of nutritional strategies and conventional therapies is the most effective for treating cancer in mice, with high potential to achieve the same in humans. My lab has begun to demonstrate the benefits of this mixed strategy for humans as well. However, the potential promise of effective drugs and stem cell–based therapies for other diseases and conditions shouldn't be an alternative to leading a life of good nutrition and other natural interventions to promote self-healing and self-preservation, since ideally drugs and more aggressive treatments should be used only when natural interventions are not enough. The reason for this is that natural interventions are the result of billions of years of evolution and in many cases can be highly coordinated and minimize or eliminate side effects, whereas drugs or other therapies will have side effects, some of which won't be detected until years after the beginning of treatment.

Statin drugs, for example, lower cholesterol by reducing the activity of the cholesterol-producing enzyme HMG-CoA reductase. But this approach is a Band-Aid solution that, instead of fixing the original problem at its source, simply reduces one of the negative symptoms *generated* by the problem. I once asked a cholesterol expert, "Why do some people's bodies produce much more cholesterol than they need? What is the body trying to do?" Both surprised and annoyed, he replied, "I don't know. It just does."

Organisms don't waste precious resources generating molecules they don't need. The right therapy for high cholesterol and cardiovascular disease is not to block generation of this molecule, but to find out what is not functioning properly in the body and what command the system is responding to when overproducing cholesterol, so that the problem can be fixed at its foundation. Simply blocking the generation of cholesterol is like adding coolant to an overheated car engine—it will undoubtedly help, but the underlying engine problem remains, and eventually the car will break down. Indeed, an analysis of eleven randomized studies found that taking statins does not change one's risk of dying.[2] The same is true for the great majority of drugs, whether they target glucose, cholesterol, or blood pressure levels: they don't fix the problem; they merely try to limit the damage it causes. Sometimes they work very well and can save or prolong lives. But often they represent a partial solution that creates new problems. This is why, as I pointed out in earlier chapters, biologists, physicians, and dietitians should work together in teams using their respective problem-solving skills to have an immediate and long-term impact on patients. My own lab has been working for years with medical doctors, and we hope this will become the clinical standard someday.

Take, for example, a forty-five-year-old person with slightly elevated cholesterol, a fifty-five-year-old man with mild hypertension, or a woman whose grandmother died of breast cancer at age eighty-five; these kinds of high risk factors can likely be reduced or reversed with a combination of the longevity diet described earlier and a periodic FMD, according to findings emerging from our clinical studies. This can forestall or even eliminate the future need for drug or stem cell therapies or may allow the use of lower levels of drugs. The major advantage of the FMD approach—compared with drug interventions and stem cell–based therapies—is that it awakens a highly coordinated response that is already built into the body but that has fallen dormant because of our steady and constant consumption of food. At present, FMD represents perhaps the safest and most potent way to reverse many age- and diet-related problems by fixing or replacing, and thereby rejuvenating, cells, systems, and organs in a natural way.

FMD achieves this by taking advantage of billions of years of evolution to activate a self-healing program resembling the embryogenesis process (i.e., the normal growth of a fetus). We have demonstrated this in mice and human cells. For example, we were able to cause severe damage and insulin deficiency in the pancreas of both mice with type 1 and type 2 diabetes and show that FMD cycles promote the regeneration of pancreatic cells to restore insulin production.[3] As described earlier in the chapter, FMD cycles also reduce fasting glucose and return prediabetic subjects to the normal glucose range. As pointed out below, in participants with normal blood pressure, glucose, cholesterol, and inflammation, we did not find big changes in the level of risk factors in response to three monthly cycles of the FMD, but we saw significant changes among those with the highest levels of risk factors before beginning the FMD. This is consistent with a rejuvenation effect—a true reversal of the physical damage or underlying problem, not simply the blockage of cholesterol synthesis or lowering of glucose levels achieved with statins or diabetes drugs.

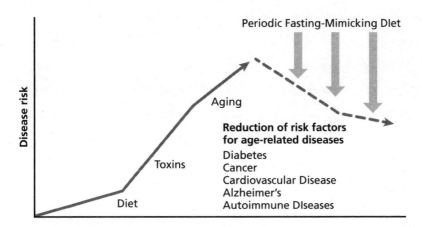

6.7. The rejuvenating effects of the FMD

The Fasting-Mimicking Diet

What follows is a simplified version of the FMD tested in our clinical study of one hundred patients at Keck Medical Center of USC and now also recommended to patients by thousands of US and UK doctors. At least ten thousand patients have undergone the ProLon FMD therapy, and there have been no reports of major side effects. The goal in this section is to provide general information that you can take to doctors and dietitians for help implementing the diet, rather than specific recipes for readers to implement on their own. The FMD clinically tested and commercialized by L-Nutra is far more complex than what I describe below, and it includes a precise formula with ingredients that cannot generally be found in stores, as well as instructions on dosages of specific ingredients based on the weight of the patient undertaking the diet. For safety and efficacy reasons, it is strongly recommended that patients do the ProLon FMD and not a "homemade" version of it, which could be ineffective and potentially harmful. L-Nutra is assembling a network of doctors and registered dietitians who specialize in these integrative therapies. Further information and resources are available at www.prolonfmd .com and on my Facebook page, @profvalterlongo. (As pointed out earlier, I do not benefit financially from the sale of ProLon.)

WHO MAY DO THE FMD

- Healthy adults in the normal weight range between the ages of eighteen and seventy years may undertake the FMD. A few genetic mutations, however, are incompatible with long-term fasting. If any side effects occur other than slight weakness, tiredness, or a headache, you should contact your doctor. Drink a small quantity of fruit juice for immediate relief.

WHO MAY NOT DO THE FMD

- Pregnant women.
- People who are underweight, have very low body mass index, or suffer from anorexia.
- People over the age of seventy, unless in superior health—and then only with a doctor's approval.
- Anyone who is fragile.
- People with liver or kidney diseases.
- People affected by pathologies, unless they have the prior approval of their specialized doctor. In the case of serious or relatively serious illnesses (cancer, diabetes, or cardiovascular, autoimmune, or neurodegenerative diseases), it is important to seek permission and approval from a disease specialist as well as from a dietitian with expertise in the FMD or in therapeutic fasting. The use of the FMD for disease treatment should for the moment be limited to clinical trials unless the doctor determines that there are no other viable options and the patient cannot wait until the conclusion of appropriate clinical trials and FDA approval.
- Patients who take medication should not undertake the FMD without the approval of their doctor with input from a dietitian or doctor who specializes in the use of the FMD. Although

it may be possible to combine the FMD with many drugs without side effects, the combination of the FMD and certain drugs could result in severe side effects.

- Patients who have low blood pressure or who are taking medication for hypertension should not undertake the FMD without the approval of a specialized doctor.
- Patients with rare genetic mutations that block the organism's capacity to produce glucose from glycerol and amino acids (gluconeogenesis).
- Athletes during training or competition. High muscular effort requires levels of glucose not available in the blood during the FMD, leading to a risk of fainting.

OTHER WARNINGS

1. The FMD can never be undertaken in association with insulin or medication that reduces sugar levels. The combination could be lethal. At the end of the FMD, the patient may still be sufficiently insulin-sensitive to have below normal levels of glucose in his or her blood. Because the use of the FMD on diabetic patients could be dangerous, we advise to do it only as part of a clinical trial. Information about upcoming clinical trials can be found on my Facebook page, @profvalterlongo.

2. Do not combine the FMD with very hot and lengthy showers, especially during hot weather. There could be a risk of fainting.

3. Drive with caution—or better yet, don't drive at all—until you know how the FMD affects you.

4. We advise undergoing the FMD in the presence of another person.

HOW OFTEN TO UNDERTAKE THE FMD

This is a decision that ideally should be made with input from a doctor or registered dietitian, but broad guidelines are as follows:

1. Once a month for overweight or obese patients with at least two risk factors for diabetes, cancer, or cardiovascular or neurodegenerative disease
2. Once every two months for average-weight patients with at least two risk factors for diabetes, cancer, or cardiovascular or neurodegenerative disease
3. Once every three months for average-weight patients with at least one risk factor for diabetes, cancer, or cardiovascular or neurodegenerative disease
4. Once every four months for healthy patients with a normal diet who are not physically active
5. Once every six months for healthy patients with an ideal diet (see chapter 4) who engage in regular physical activity

WHEN TO START THE FMD

■ Many people decide to start FMD on a Sunday night so they can end the following Friday night. This decision is based purely on social considerations, allowing them to return to the transition diet on Friday night and to a normal diet on Saturday night.

■ For at least one week before the FMD, we recommend follow-ing the Longevity Diet, with 0.36 grams of protein per pound of body weight per day, preferably obtained from vegetables and fish. Multivitamin supplements of omega-3 should be taken at least twice during this preparatory week (see chapter 4).

The FMD

Day 1 1,100 calories	• 500 calories from complex carbohydrates (vegetables such as broccoli, tomatoes, carrots, pumpkin, mushrooms, etc.) • 500 calories from healthy fats (nuts, olive oil) • 1 multivitamin and mineral supplement • 1 omega-3/omega-6 supplement • Sugarless tea (up to 3 to 4 cups per day) • 25 grams of plant-based protein, mainly from nuts • Unlimited water
Days 2–5 800 calories	• 400 calories from complex carbohydrates (vegetables such as broccoli, tomatoes, carrots, pumpkin, mushrooms, etc.) • 400 calories from healthy fats (nuts, olive oil) • 1 multivitamin and mineral supplement • 1 omega-3/omega-6 supplement • Sugarless tea (up to 3 to 4 cups per day) • Unlimited water
The above components can be divided between breakfast, lunch, and dinner, or they can be taken as two meals and a snack.	
Day 6 Transition diet	For 24 hours following the end of the five-day FMD, patients should follow a diet based on complex carbohydrates (vegetables, cereals, pasta, rice, bread, fruit, etc.), and minimize the consumption of fish, meat, saturated fats, pastries, cheeses, milk, etc.

WHAT TO EXPECT

SIDE EFFECTS

1. Some people feel weak during parts of the FMD. Others say they feel more energetic.

2. Some patients complain of light- or average-intensity head-aches. This effect is usually greatly reduced by day 4 or 5, and eliminated entirely by the second or third FMD cycle.

3. Most people feel hungry during the first few days of the FMD. This effect is greatly reduced by day 4 or 5 and on all days during the second or third FMD cycle.

4. Some people suffer a slight backache that disappears once they resume a normal diet.

POSITIVE EFFECTS

In addition to the production of stem cells, the reduction of abdominal fat, and lower levels of risk factors for various illnesses, many people report the following beneficial effects during or after FMD:

1. Glowing skin, which many describe as "younger looking."
2. Stronger mental focus.
3. An ability to resist bingeing once they resume a normal diet. Many reduce their consumption of sugar and calories, and are less prone to excess in their consumption of coffee, alcohol, desserts, etc.

Now that you understand the Longevity Diet and how and why it works, and the basics of the FMD, I will go into detail in the following chapters on how this program can have profound effects when it comes to preventing, delaying, treating, and even reversing specific diseases. The next five chapters contain more detailed information on the work I and my fellow researchers and physicians around the world are conducting into the potent links between diet and disease, and they are especially intended to help those individuals at high risk for or suffering from cancer, diabetes, cardiovascular disease, neurodegenerative disorders (especially Alzheimer's), and autoimmune diseases. It is my hope that this book can help as many people as possible take control of their health so that they can supplement the standard care they are receiving with this integrative, inexpensive approach. First up, some remarkable results involving cancer.

Chapter 7

Nutrition and Fasting-Mimicking Diets in Cancer Prevention and Treatment*

[For their review of this chapter, I thank Tanya Dorff, oncologist and associate professor of clinical medicine, USC Norris Comprehensive Cancer Center; Alessio Nencioni, associate professor and doctor of internal medicine and geriatrics, University of Genova San Martino Hospital; and Alessandro Laviano, professor of clinical medicine, Sapienza University, Rome.]

The Magic Shield

My graduate school training and research in pathology, immunology, and neurobiology was "translational"—meaning, I focused on turning basic scientific discoveries into medical therapies for humans. With this as my goal, fifteen years ago I decided to switch

---

* The contents of this chapter must not be used in self-diagnosis or the self-administration of therapies. This information is intended for medical professionals following your disease.

a large part of my lab to clinical research. As I mentioned in chapter 2, I was motivated by my experiences with children suffering from cancer at Children's Hospital Los Angeles. The medical community, I realized, had a deep understanding of how DNA and cellular damage affect cancer cells, but almost no knowledge of how to protect normal cells, which was the focus of my lab.

Our first cancer-related mouse study, as mentioned in chapter 2, was very simple—basically a spin-off of our studies with microorganisms.

Paola Fabrizio, a postdoctoral fellow researcher in my group, and I coauthored a series of papers on studies using yeast as a model organism to identify what genes accelerate the aging process. Mario Mirisola, another researcher in my laboratory, helped me identify the links between genes that accelerate aging and make cells more vulnerable, and specific nutrients. Remarkably, the genes that made the cells weaker were the same genes central to cancer—the oncogenes.

Here's how the process works: When certain genes in cancer cells are modified through a mutation (a change in the DNA sequence), they become oncogenes. This change lets cancer cells divide more than they should, regardless of the signals they receive to stop dividing. We discovered that oncogenes also make cells weaker and more vulnerable to the damage caused by toxins. This occurs because these same oncogenes give cells a key characteristic: the ability to disobey orders and continue growing.

When I began my cancer studies, every researcher was looking for a magic bullet that would seek out and destroy only cancer cells. I don't remember when I first dreamed up the idea, but I remember calling one of my colleagues, a famous aging researcher, to float my theory: "I think I've figured out a way to distinguish all cancer cells from all normal cells," I told her. "It's not a magic bullet—it's a magic *shield*."

I don't think she had any idea what I was talking about.

What I proposed, and eventually called "differential stress resistance," was based on the idea that if you starve an organism, it will go into a highly protected, nongrowth mode—this is "the shield." But a cancer cell will disobey this order and continue growing even when it is starved, because the oncogene is stuck in an "always on" mode.

Imagine a battlefield where ancient Romans and Carthaginians are mixed together wearing very similar uniforms. The common approach of cancer therapies is to seek a magic "arrow" (or "bullet") that will kill only the Carthaginian soldiers, without harming the Romans. This is tricky, because the soldiers all look the same to archers standing fifty yards away.

But suppose before shooting their arrows, the archers ordered the soldiers, in Latin, to kneel and raise their shields. Because only the Romans would understand the command, they would take cover, while the Carthaginians would remain standing, exposed to the incoming arrows.

In this imaginary historical example, the Romans are the normal cells of the body, the Carthaginians the cancer cells, the archers the oncologists, and the arrows the chemotherapy. If you starve a cancer patient before injecting chemotherapy, normal cells will respond by putting up a defensive shield. But the cancer cells will ignore the command to kneel and thus remain vulnerable—providing a way to potentially eradicate cancer cells with minimal damage to normal cells.

When I first proposed starving cancer patients, oncologists thought it was a very bad idea. Because cancer patients often lose weight during chemotherapy, oncologists instruct them to eat more, not less. Clearly, we needed very convincing results in mice before we would get approval for a clinical trial with human subjects.

I asked Changhan Lee, one of my graduate students in the Los Angeles laboratory, and Lizzia Raffaghello, a researcher in Genoa, to perform a simple experiment: switch mice with cancer to a water-only diet for two or three days before giving them multiple cycles of chemotherapy.

The results were stunning: virtually all the fasting mice were alive and moving around normally after high-dose chemotherapy. Mice on a normal diet, however, were sick and moving very little after chemotherapy. In the following weeks, 65 percent of the mice that did not fast died, whereas nearly all the fasted mice survived. We reproduced this same effect using a wide variety of chemotherapy drugs. As hoped and predicted, starvation consistently caused "multi-stress resistance," or protection against many different toxins in normal cells, but not cancer cells. We now knew this approach had great clinical potential, but it still would not be easy getting the medical community to give it a chance.

A Note to Animal Activists

This seems like a good place to say a word about animal testing. From time to time I receive emails from animal rights activists asking why mice must suffer and die for the sake of research.

Here is my answer:

First, we do as much of our work as possible with cells and microorganisms, not mice. However, before any human clinical trial can begin, we have no choice but to test interventions in mice.

Regarding the supposed cruelty of a forced fast, it's worth noting that mice, like humans, are perfectly capable of going without food for a few days. Indeed, they benefit from fasting—with longer, healthier, less disease-prone lives. It's true that when we give the mice chemotherapy, they suffer. I am troubled by this fact. It seems morally wrong. But I don't see any alternative.

We confine our animal studies to the minimum required in the lead-up to human clinical trials. In almost every case, these studies target advanced-stage diseases either deadly or devastating to patients.

A few years ago, I responded to a letter from an animal activist with the following question: "If your child, sister, or father was dying, and the only treatment that might save his/her life needed to be tested first in mice, would you condone the mouse experiments? Or would you choose to see your loved one die?"

I know many activists will still object, but I ask that they be honest and consider the consequences. If they don't condone animal experiments under any circumstances, even those necessary to develop treatments for deadly diseases, then they should never take any drug—even aspirin or antibiotics—and tell their family members to do the same.

I believe animal experiments should be undertaken only as a precursor to human clinical trials in the treatment of advanced-stage and major illnesses. In the absence of better options, these trials are, unfortunately, a necessary evil.

Curing Cancer (in Mice)

Here's another military scenario with parallels to fighting cancer: In 1812, Napoleon invaded Russia with more than 450,000 men. As the French army moved toward Moscow, the Russian forces didn't fight. They retreated, burning their own villages and towns before the enemy's advance.

Napoleon was surprised and confused. The invasion had started in June, but the Russians refused to fight until December. The strategic retreat was meant to weaken the French army. By winter, Napoleon's army was in tatters after enduring months of starvation, freezing conditions, and the final attack by the Russians. When the war ended, 400,000 French soldiers had perished.

Cancer cells behave like Napoleon's army, advancing even when it would be wiser to stop. To stay alive, they require a lot of nourishment. The typical nutritional recommendation given by doctors to cancer patients is to "eat well," and sometimes to "eat more than normal." This makes intuitive sense, as it made intuitive sense for the Russian army to engage Napoleon's invaders the moment they arrived, in the summer of 1812, when they were well fed. But because the Russians waited until the French soldiers were at their weakest, the combination of cold, starvation, and targeted attacks by the Russians defeated them permanently. In the same way, starved cancer cells are most vulnerable to the assault of chemotherapy after fasting.

Having conceived the idea of a starvation-induced magic shield, I remembered a basic lesson from evolutionary biology:

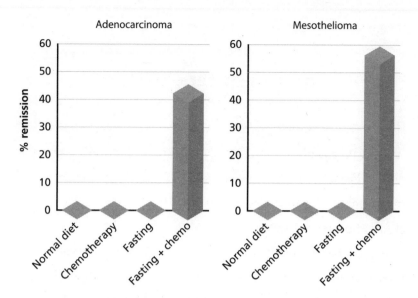

7.1. *Percentage of lung cancer remission in mice subjected to the FMD with and without chemotherapy*[1]

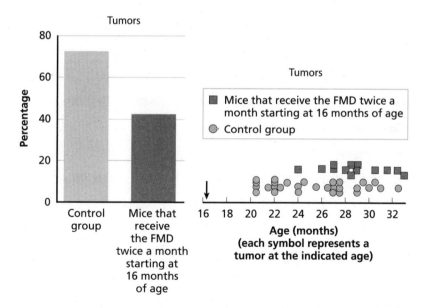

7.2. *Cycles of FMD reduce and delay cancer in mice*

the great majority of genetic mutations (changes in the DNA) are deleterious, but their negative consequences usually appear only under certain conditions. Abundant mutations in the DNA sequence of cancer cells may well increase their ability to grow, but those same mutations will greatly impede the cancer cell's ability to survive in challenging environments, for example under the double onslaught of starvation and chemotherapy.

Could this theoretical scenario actually work? Our animal studies and those of other researchers show that fasting, in addition to protecting normal cells, makes chemotherapy much more toxic to melanoma, breast cancer, prostate cancer, lung cancer, colorectal cancer, neuroblastoma, and many other cancers. In many cases, cycles of fasting (or of a fasting-mimicking diet) are as effective as chemotherapy at fighting cancer. However, neither strategy alone is optimal. Permanent therapeutic effects are achieved only through the combination of fasting and chemotherapy. In mouse studies, we saw fasting combined with chemotherapy definitively cured cancer even in the disease's end stages, after it had metastasized. Not all mice were cured, but we and others regularly obtained a 20 to 60 percent cure rate for a variety of cancers.

FMD and Immune-System-Dependent Killing of Cancer Cells

Among new therapies to treat and, in some cases, cure cancer, perhaps the most promising is immunotherapy, which relies on the immune system to kill cancer cells. In another very promising study at USC, we showed that FMD can trigger the same effects produced by immunotherapy.[2] The study, which looked at breast cancer and skin cancer cells, found that FMD performs two main functions: (1) it weakens cancer cells and removes the protective shield safeguarding them from immune cells; and (2) it renews and revs the immune system, making it more aggressive toward the cancer.[3]

FMD and Chemotherapy-Related Steroids

Corticosteroids such as prednisolone, methylprednisolone, and dexamethasone are frequently used in combination with chemotherapy in cancer treatment. In a recent publication, we showed that the corticosteroid dexamethasone increased the toxicity to mice of the chemotherapy drug doxorubicin by increasing the level of glucose in the blood.[4] In earlier chapters, I described how glucose accelerates aging in cells but also makes them weaker when exposed to toxins. Thus, by increasing the levels of blood glucose, corticosteroids make normal cells in mice weaker while probably making cancer cells stronger. This effect was reversed by adding the fasting-mimicking diet to the dexamethasone and chemotherapy treatment. Thus, our results indicate that corticosteroids should never be combined with chemotherapy unless there is no viable alternative. In fact, high glucose levels in combination with chemotherapy in patients are associated with an increased risk of developing infections and with higher death rates when compared with patients with normal blood glucose.[5] Thus, both our mouse data and preliminary clinical data indicate that steroid hormones that increase blood glucose levels can be detrimental in combination with chemotherapy.

Fasting and Fasting-Mimicking Diets in Human Cancer Treatment

After the 2008 publication of our first study on the powerful, protective effect of fasting on mice exposed to chemotherapy, the press was abuzz with stories on a fasting-dependent "magic shield" with the potential to protect cancer patients. One such article in the *Los Angeles Times* caught the eye of a local judge, Nora Quinn, who had recently been diagnosed with breast cancer and was about to undergo chemotherapy. Shortly after the story appeared, one of the judge's friends called me at USC and informed me that Quinn had been fasting for eight days. I was horrified. "That's crazy," I said. "Please tell your friend to start eating immediately."

As the news reached patients, many decided to improvise and came up with their own dangerous versions of the FMD. Luckily for Quinn, she ended up responding well to shorter periods of fasting in combination with chemotherapy, and didn't suffer many of the treatment's debilitating side effects. I'm happy to report that when I recently communicated with her, she remained cancer-free.

Another early adopter of FMD was Air France pilot Jean-Jacques Trochon. Diagnosed with metastatic kidney cancer and multiple masses in the lungs, he had read about our mouse studies in the news and contacted me seeking advice on fasting before chemotherapy. Working with his oncologist, Trochon followed all my instructions with disciplined rigor to combine an FMD with a plant-based therapy developed by another scientist. Two years later, he was cancer-free and had returned to flying.

These anecdotes aren't proof that the combination of anticancer therapy and FMD cures some cancers. But together with the mouse and the clinical data, they point to a potentially effective strategy for improving conventional treatment options while reducing side effects.

After we published the 2008 fasting and chemotherapy mouse study, emails started pouring in from cancer patients interested in trying FMD. I put a young physician working in my laboratory in charge of following up and communicating with these patients' oncologists.

In our initial interactions with clinical oncologists, we were not taken seriously. But we had compared the effects of fasting with the chemotherapy drug of choice in the treatment of various cancers. We knew that combining the two had produced a synergic boost in efficacy, at least in mice.

We called the oncologists of each patient who had contacted us. Some wouldn't return our calls. In several cases, my researcher showed up at the clinic to personally request copies of the patients' files. Eventually we collected data on ten patients: seven women and three men, between the ages of forty-four and seventy-eight, diagnosed with different types and stages of cancer:

Demographical and Clinical Information of Patients

	Gender	Age	Primary neoplasia	Stage at diagnosis
Case 1	Female	51	Breast	IIA
Case 2	Male	68	Esophagus	IVB
Case 3	Male	74	Prostate	II
Case 4	Female	61	Lung (NSCLC)	IV
Case 5	Female	74	Uterus	IV
Case 6	Female	44	Ovary	IA
Case 7	Male	66	Prostate	IV/DI
Case 8	Female	51	Breast	IIA
Case 9	Female	48	Breast	IIA
Case 10	Female	78	Breast	IIA

7.3. *Personal and clinical data of ten patients involved in the study focused on fasting and chemotherapy combination*

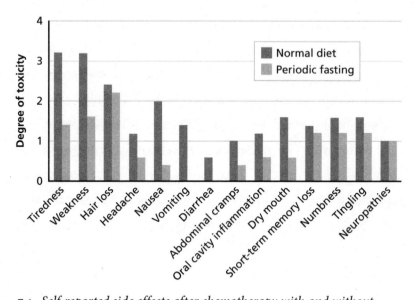

7.4. *Self-reported side effects after chemotherapy with and without fasting*

Each of these patients had voluntarily fasted for 48 to 140 hours prior to and 5 to 56 hours following chemotherapy. They had received an average of four cycles of various chemotherapy drugs in combination with fasting. None reported significant side effects caused by the fasting itself, other than hunger and light-headedness. Six patients who underwent chemotherapy both with and without fasting reported a reduction in fatigue, weakness, and gastrointestinal side effects while fasting. In patients whose cancer progression could be assessed, fasting did not impede the chemotherapy-induced reduction of tumor volume or tumor markers.

Since then, several other clinical studies have followed.

Clinical Trials

In collaboration with oncologists at the USC Norris Comprehensive Cancer Center, we performed a clinical trial with eighteen patients on a water-only fast of 24, 48, and 72 hours' duration before receiving platinum-based chemotherapy.[6] Below are the results. In terms of side effects caused by chemotherapy, 72-hour fasting was generally associated with more protection than 24-hour fasting was. However, the water-only fasting was so difficult for patients that it took over 5 years to complete this small study. This limitation led to funding by the National Cancer Institute of the US National Institutes of Health to develop a FMD specific for cancer (see below).

Toxicity	24 hours # (%) N = 6	48 hours # (%) N = 7	72 hours # (%) N = 7
Constitutional / General			
Fatigue Grade 1 or 2	6 (100%)	5 (71%)	6 (86%)
Alopecia Grade 1	6 (100%)	5 (71%)	7 (100%)
Gastrointestinal			
Nausea Grade 1 or 2	6 (100%)	6 (86%)	3 (43%)
Vomiting Grade 1 or 2	5 (83%)	3 (43%)	0
Constipation Grade 1 or 2	3 (50%)	2 (28%)	3 (43%)
Diarrhea Grade 1 or 2	2 (33%)	0	4 (57%)
Hematologic			
Neutropenia Grade 1 or 2	1 (17%)	3 (43%)	1 (14%)
Neutropenia Grade 3 or 4	4 (67%)	1 (14%)	2 (29%)
Thrombocytopenia Grade 1 or 2	4 (67%)	1 (14%)	1 (14%)
Laboratory / Metabolic			
Hyponatremia (Low serum sodium) Grade 1	1 (17%)	1 (14%)	1 (14%)
Hyponatremia Grade 3	1 (17%)	0	0
Hypokalemia (Low serum potassium) Grade 1	1 (17%)	2 (28%)	0
Hyperglycemia (Low serum glucose) Grade 1 or 2	4 (67%)	1 (14%)	0
Elevated AST/ALT Grade 1	4 (67%)	0	3 (43%)
Neurologic			
Peripheral Neuropathy Grade 1	3 (50%)	1 (14%)	1 (14%)
Dizziness Grade 1 or 2	1 (17%)	5 (71%)	2 (29%)

7.5. Different protective effects of fasting for 24, 48, and 72 hours against side effects of platinum-based chemotherapy in breast, ovarian, uterine, and pulmonary cancer patients

Leiden University in Holland also published a small, random-ized clinical trial of thirteen patients undergoing two days of water-only fasting compared with a control group.[7] The study is also consistent with the protective benefits of fasting with respect to chemotherapy side effects.

Finally, a study at Charité–University Medicine Berlin tested the impact of a very low-calorie FMD in thirty-four women with breast and ovarian cancer. Each woman received multiple cycles of chemotherapy either with or without fasting. Those on the FMD experienced a clear reduction in the side effects caused by chemotherapy. That study has not yet been published.

Ongoing clinical trials involving more than three hundred patients are currently testing the efficacy of a four-day FMD in combination with standard cancer therapy. Centers involved in these trials include the Mayo Clinic, the USC Norris Comprehensive Cancer Center, Leiden University Medical Center, and the University of Genova San Martino Hospital. An additional ten European and US hospitals are committed to begin similar trials once funds become available.

FMD AND CANCER THERAPY: CLINICAL EVIDENCE AND GUIDELINES FOR ONCOLOGISTS AND CANCER PATIENTS

- Extensive animal testing from at least six independent laboratories shows the efficacy of fasting or FMD in protecting against the side effects caused by a wide range of chemotherapy drugs.

- Extensive animal testing from at least six independent laboratories shows the efficacy of fasting or FMD in increasing the effect of standard therapy on breast cancer, prostate cancer, colorectal cancer, pancreatic cancer, neuroblastoma, glioma, lung cancer, mesothelioma, melanoma, and others.

- Three completed small clinical trials and one case series report involving seventy-five patients provide initial evidence that fasting and FMD are safe and potentially effective in protecting patients from multiple side effects of chemotherapy.
- Ongoing clinical trials on Chemolieve at leading cancer centers, which have now tested over two hundred patients, provide additional evidence for the safety and potentially protective effect of the FMD against chemotherapy side effects.

The FMD product for cancer patients, Chemolieve, can be recommended to patients by their oncologists once additional tests are done and if the results are positive. Until this product is shown to be effective and comes to market, the FMD remains an unproven method of cancer treatment and should be considered preferably as part of clinical trials and only in combination with standard-of-care therapies under medical supervision. The patient should be informed of the risks of undergoing a support therapy that is not yet fully tested. Following are my FMD recommendations to oncologists and cancer patients:

1. If the oncologist agrees, the patient may fast or adopt an FMD for three days before and one day after receiving chemotherapy or other standard-of-care drugs. Depending on the type of chemotherapy being administered and the interval between cycles, this regimen could change. Patients should hold off on resuming their regular diet until the chemotherapy is below toxic blood levels (usually 24 to 48 hours after administration). For treatment lasting up to three days, patients can adopt an FMD one day prior to, three days during, and one

day after chemotherapy for a total of five days. Longer treatment periods, while difficult to integrate with fasting, may still be combined with a higher-calorie FMD with the oncologist's approval.

2. We have rarely seen major side effects caused by FMDs, and all occurred when people made their own fasting or FMD; one patient showed an increase in liver toxicity markers while doing her own fast while receiving a chemo cocktail. Several patients fainted while taking hot showers after multiple days of fasting—probably because of the reduction in blood pressure and glucose levels. Another FMD-related risk: resuming regular eating habits immediately following chemotherapy could cause liver damage due to the combination of hepatotoxic drugs and the proliferation of liver cells. For this reason, it is important to wait a minimum of 24 hours after the chemotherapy is administered before resuming a normal diet.

3. While most people can safely drive or operate machinery while fasting, a few will be impaired. When in doubt, avoid both activities during the fasting period.

4. Starting 24 hours after chemotherapy, the patient should eat only rice, pasta, bread or a similar source of carbohydrates, vegetables, and vegetable soups, and some fruit for a full 24 hours. Then a normal diet can be resumed, paying particular attention to nourishment (vitamins, minerals, protein, and essential fats).

5. The patient should try to return to regular body weight before undertaking another fasting cycle.

6. With regard to weight loss caused by fasting, obese patients

should consult their personal physician on the advisability of maintaining their new weight or regaining what they lost.

7. Diabetic patients should not undergo fasting unless it is approved by their diabetologist or endocrinologist.

8. Patients should not fast while taking metformin, insulin, or similar drugs.

9. Patients on hypertension medication should speak to their doctor about blood-pressure drops caused by fasting and the risk of combining fasting with medications.

10. Until clinical trials are completed, fasting will remain an experimental procedure and should be considered only with the approval of a patient's oncologist in combination with standard-of-care therapies, preferably as part of a clinical trial and when other options are not available or are known to be ineffective.

11. Between fasting cycles, we recommend that cancer patients maintain a low-sugar, mostly plant-based, low-protein but otherwise high-nourishment diet which allow them to maintain a healthy weight and normal BMI. A registered dietitian should be consulted to avoid malnourishment and unwanted weight loss (see the Longevity Diet in chapter 4).

Nutrition and FMD for Cancer Prevention

Although the Longevity Diet (see chapter 4) can be generally applied for cancer prevention, it has the potential to be especially beneficial for people with certain genetic mutations—such as the BRCA genes—which put them at a greatly increased risk of cancer. Prophylactic mastectomies and other surgical procedures can

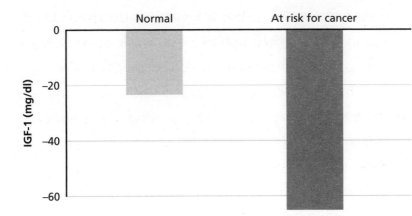

7.6. Insulin-like growth factor-1, associated with cancer and aging, is reduced more effectively, after three cycles of FMD in individuals at risk for cancer (>225, or with IGF-1 levels above 225 ng/mL at the beginning of the trial)

reduce the incidence of genetically induced cancers, but nutrition and FMD may also help. Dietary interventions additionally have the potential to reduce the chance of recurrence in previously diagnosed patients whose cancer is in remission. It is important to stress that patients should not attempt to replace prophylactic mastectomies with nutritional interventions whose efficacy remains to be established.

BELOW ARE DIETARY RECOMMENDATIONS FOR PEOPLE AT HIGH RISK FOR CANCER:

1. Follow the Longevity Diet, described in chapter 4, with protein intake reduced to the lower range of about 0.31 grams per pound of body weight per day.

2. Limit fish intake to one or two times a week; otherwise stick to plant-based foods.

3. Reduce sugars to very low levels. Also minimize the con-

sumption of pasta and breads. It is important to keep blood-sugar levels as low as possible within the safe range.

4. Maintain a healthy weight and BMI (see chapter 4).

5. Exercise regularly (see chapter 5).

6. Undergo a five-day FMD every one to three months, depending on your weight and health status (once every three to six months if you are very healthy with ideal weight and abdominal fat; once every month if you are overweight or obese and at high risk for cancer). Remember that in mouse studies, FMD was as effective as chemotherapy against cancer. Instead of damaging normal tissues and organs, it protected them.

7. Nourish yourself with essential fatty acids (omega-3 and omega-6), vitamins, and minerals from a variety of vegetables (broccoli, carrots, green peppers, tomatoes, garbanzo beans, lentils, peas, black beans, etc.) and fish (salmon, anchovies). Your immune system is one of the major defenses against cancer. The diet must be balanced to kill cancerous or precancerous cells without causing deficiencies in your immune system or hormonal changes that can make you frail. See the high-nourishment diet examples at the end of this book.

8. Discuss with your oncologist the option of taking 6 grams of vitamin C or Ester-C® daily for a few weeks every 6 months. Multiple studies have demonstrated vitamin C to possess cancer-fighting properties, although its effectiveness in preventing cancer is controversial. Either way, vitamin C taken for a few weeks every 6 months at this level is not known to have major side effects, and the patient and doctor could con-

sider continuing high-level vitamin C consumption for longer periods.

9. Consume plenty of good fats from olive oil, nuts, and fish, but minimize saturated fats, even those that are vegetable-derived.

10. Consume as little alcohol as possible.

Our clinical trials looking into FMD and cancer prevention and treatment are ongoing, but if early results are any indication, it could be a powerful new weapon in the arsenal we have to fight, and one day defeat, cancer. Next up, a look at our studies into FMD and diabetes.

Chapter 8

Nutrition, FMD, and Diabetes Prevention and Treatment*

[For their review of this chapter, I thank Hanno Pijl, endocrinologist, diabetologist, and director of the Clinic for Endocrinology and Metabolic Disease at Leiden University, and Clayton Frenzel, bariatric surgeon.]

Type 2 Diabetes

Type 2 diabetes, by far the most common of the two types, affects more than 27 million people in the United States; an additional 86 million people have prediabetes, meaning they have elevated risk factors for diabetes. According to the World Health Organization, the number of people diagnosed with diabetes globally has more than quadrupled in the past thirty-five years, from 100 mil-

---

* The contents of this chapter must not be used in self-diagnosis or the self-administration of therapies. This information is intended for medical professionals following your disease.

lion in 1980 to 422 million in 2014. The disease is diagnosed by measuring the average level of glucose in the blood (by an HbA1c test), or by detecting glucose levels above 125 mg/dL after an overnight fast—this latter measure is known as one's "fasting glucose level." Typical symptoms include high thirst, frequent urination, blurry vision, irritability, numbness of the hands or feet, and fatigue.

In type 2 diabetes, the pancreas produces insulin, but muscle cells, liver cells, and fat cells do not respond properly to it. When cells become insulin-resistant, glucose accumulates in the blood. You can think of insulin as the key needed to unlock the gate that lets glucose enter the cells, but also the key that closes the door that allows glucose to be released by the liver. In type 2 diabetic patients, that key isn't working properly, the gate doesn't open completely, and glucose cannot enter cells at the normal rate.

But the damage to normal cells begins well before diabetes is diagnosed. People who are obese or overweight with high levels of abdominal fat have a far greater chance of developing diabetes and prediabetes (when fasting glucose levels are between 100 and 125 mg/dL).

The risk for diabetes is sixfold higher among women with body mass index (BMI) of 25 than those with a BMI of 21. For a five-foot-five-inch-tall woman, this is the difference between weighing 154 pounds and 130 pounds. A similar effect is observed in men with a BMI of 27.5 and 22, which indicates that a five-foot-eight-inch-tall male weighing 152 pounds would have a risk for diabetes that is five times lower than that of a man of the same height weighing 191 pounds (see fig. 8.1).[1]

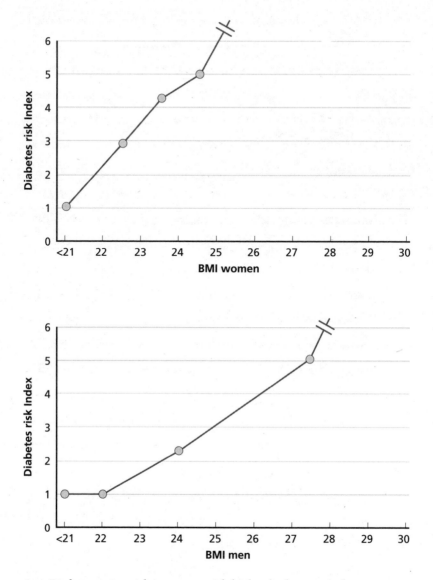

8.1. *Diabetes onset risk increases with higher body mass index*

Another study indicates the best way to assess risk for diabetes is by measuring abdominal fat via waist circumference. Men with a waist measurement above forty inches and women with a waist measurement above thirty-four inches are at the highest risk.[2]

Nutrition, Weight Management, and Diabetes Prevention

Maintaining an ideal weight will minimize the chance of developing diabetes. We know from both human and monkey studies that a severely calorie-restricted diet can either completely prevent diabetes, as in monkeys, or, as in humans, cause such a dramatic reduction in fasting glucose levels and abdominal fat that it would be highly unlikely that these individuals would develop diabetes.[3]

However, the great majority of people cannot maintain a 30 percent calorie-restricted diet, and don't want to give up most of the foods they enjoy; nor should they want to lose large quantities of muscle mass or become too thin, which would be unavoidable after prolonged calorie restriction. Also, several studies indicate calorie restriction does not reduce fasting glucose among obese people the same way it does among people starting from a normal weight.[4] To prevent diabetes, then, it is important to identify strategies better suited to a majority of people.

In the following section, I present both the everyday dietary changes and the periodic fasting-mimicking diets that can be adopted to prevent and help reverse diabetes.

The Longevity Diet for Diabetes Prevention and Potential Reversal

Adopting the Longevity Diet described in chapter 4 can help prevent and has the potential to reverse diabetes in some subjects.

Not only will it help you maintain or reach a healthy weight and abdominal fat level—especially when combined with the exercise guidelines in chapter 5—but also it may reduce diabetes incidence independently of weight. Here are specific dietary interventions that can help prevent and treat diabetes:

1. Eat within twelve hours or fewer per day.

   In chapter 4, I discussed the research related to a healthy time period for daily eating. A five-foot-two woman weighing 154 pounds who normally eats breakfast at 8 a.m. and has a late-night snack at 11 p.m. is eating for fifteen hours a day. This probably affects her weight and possibly her sleep.[5] One simple strategy for dropping to a healthier weight is to reduce the eating period to eleven or twelve hours per day—in the above example, this would mean eating the last snack by 7 or 8 p.m.

   This technique can be adjusted to further regulate weight. For example, if limiting food intake to eleven to twelve hours per day isn't sufficient, it can be limited to ten or even eight hours per day (8 a.m. to 6 p.m., or 8 a.m. to 4 p.m.), although limiting the food intake period to less than eleven to twelve hours could have side effects including gallstones. Furthermore, a number of studies indicate that skipping breakfast could have a negative effect on overall health and increase cardiovascular disease.[6] However, restricting food intake to an eleven- to twelve-hour window every day is often observed in very long-lived populations, so this more permissive time frame is probably a safer choice until further studies become available.

2. Be nourished: eat more, not less, but better.

As discussed in chapter 4, if you ate 5.3 ounces of pasta or pizza with 5.3 ounces of cheese, you could be consuming 1,100 calories in a relatively small portion that is deficient in important vitamins and minerals. If you instead ate 1.4 ounces of pasta (about 140 calories) and an additional 14 ounces of garbanzo beans (about 330 calories) plus 11 ounces of mixed vegetables (about 210 calories) and 0.5 ounce of olive oil (about 120 calories), you would reach only 800 calories, while eating a large portion rich in proteins, healthy fats, complex carbohydrates, vitamins, and minerals.

Option A (wrong choice)
5.3 oz. pasta (540 calories) + 5.3 oz. cheese (550 calories) + 2 oz. sauce (20 calories)

Option B (right choice)
1.4 oz. pasta (about 140 calories) + 14 oz. garbanzo beans (soaked

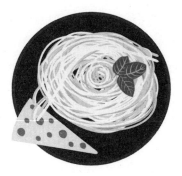 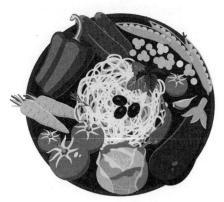

8.2. *Option A = 12.6 ounces,* *Option B = 27 ounces, 800 calories*
1,110 calories

and drained, about 330 calories) + 11 oz. mixed vegetables (about 210 calories) + 0.5 oz. olive oil (120 calories)

Option B is obviously a better choice, for multiple reasons:

- Option B provides enough proteins and more vitamins, minerals, healthy fats, and other nutrients, which can nourish and signal satiety to the brain.
- It causes a lower release of insulin.
- It requires eating food weighing more than twice as much as Option A, therefore filling and expanding the stomach and sending the brain additional signals of satiety, while providing 30 percent fewer calories.
- It replaces the bad saturated animal fats contained in cheese with the protective monounsaturated fats contained in olive oil.
- For many people, Option B will eventually even taste better than Option A, because saturated fats and sugars tend to cover the flavor of other ingredients.
- Many will also feel lighter and avoid acid reflux or heartburn, despite having eaten twice as much food. Of course, some people consuming large meals, particularly at night, may experience acid reflux even if a meal like Option B is consumed. In this case, it's best to talk to a specialized doctor and reduce your meal size.

3. Eat two meals a day plus a snack.

As also noted in chapter 4, eating small meals five or six times a day is generally a bad idea, particularly for people who are gaining unwanted weight or needing to lose weight.

The ideal strategy to maintain or lose weight is to eat a light breakfast plus lunch and then have a snack or very light meal for dinner, as is the norm in several very long-lived populations. The other option is to have a light breakfast, a snack for lunch, and a larger dinner.

Note that for some people, especially older and sick people, one large meal per day may cause indigestion or acid reflux, in which case it may be necessary to move the larger meal to earlier in the day or go back to breakfast plus two smaller meals per day instead of one larger one. If in doubt and if at all possible, you can consult with a dietitian to determine the best strategy.

4. Maximize complex carbohydrates (whole grains, vegetables, legumes); reduce pasta, rice, and bread; and minimize sugar and bad fat.

Even once you reach an ideal weight and waist circumference, the levels of sugars or starches (rice, pasta, bread, soft drinks, etc.) as well as the levels of saturated fats (cheese, butter, candy, etc.) must be minimized. The liver uses excess sugars to generate fats, which can be stored there or transported to various storage sites including the abdomen (visceral fat) and to areas under the skin throughout the body (subcutaneous fat).

The role of fat intake in obesity and diseases is very controversial. In the past, it was commonly believed that a high-fat diet leads to obesity. We now know that while a high-fat diet can also contribute to obesity, it's a high-sugar, high-starch diet that deserves a lot of the blame.

As for a high-fat, low-carbohydrate diet, while it's true

that in most cases this regimen will result in weight loss, a significant portion of that loss comes from water and muscle. In addition, the high-fat and high-protein diet, in the long run, is the worst of all possible regimens both in terms of overall mortality and the incidence of cancer or death from cancer (see chapter 4).

Good fats—particularly those coming from olive oil and nuts (walnuts, almonds, hazelnuts)—have been consistently associated with health and longevity. Consume a handful of nuts every day and pour olive oil generously on salads and other dishes.

5. Adopt a low but sufficient protein diet.

Although obesity is known to increase one's risk of diabetes, protein intake may be just as big of a factor. One study following forty thousand men for up to twenty years showed a twofold increased risk for diabetes associated with a low-carbohydrate, high-protein diet.[7] Those results are consistent with our 2014 study of six thousand people in the United States indicating increased diabetes risk in those with the highest protein intake, although the small population size limited the significance of our results.[8]

Two of our papers we published in 2011 and 2015 studied diseases in one hundred Laron syndrome patients living in Ecuador. Because of the mutation in the growth hormone receptor gene (GHR), they experience dwarfism and become obese at a higher rate than their relatives who live in the same communities and eat the same diet but do not have Laron syndrome. Even though obesity is one of the major risk factors for diabetes, not one of the Laron subjects in Ecuador has developed diabetes. Because proteins are the major regulators of the growth hormone gene, these results are in agreement with the papers discussed above, and similarly suggest that high protein intake may promote diabetes in part by increasing the activity of growth hormone and the growth factor IGF-1, associated at high levels with multiple diseases.

The absence of growth hormone receptor (which can be viewed as having an effect similar to that of eating a very low-protein diet) eliminates or reduces drastically obesity's causal effect on diabetes. In fact, mice with defects in the growth hormone receptor are also protected from diabetes—results that support our conclusions in humans. The strongest proof for our hypothesis came in 2015, when we measured glucose tolerance in the Laron syndrome group. Far from being insulin-resistant, they turned out to be insulin-sensitive, meaning their insulin worked better than normal even in overweight or obese individuals.[9] Because insulin resistance is the key cause of diabetes, this insight may explain why none of the Ecuador Laron patients have yet developed this metabolic disease.

The above recommendations for preventing diabetes may also be beneficial for treatment of the disease, although, as with the cancer recommendations, further studies are necessary to demonstrate this effect.

FASTING AND FASTING-MIMICKING DIETS IN DIABETES TREATMENT

5:2 Diet

Two major short-term interventions involving some form of fasting have been demonstrated to be effective against multiple diabetes risk factors (excluding interventions that use severe calorie restriction lasting weeks to months). One of them is the periodic FMD developed by my laboratory. The other, developed by Dr. Michelle Harvie of the University of Manchester—and subsequently modified and popularized as the "5:2" diet by doctor and journalist Michael Mosley—involved overweight subjects who, for two days a week during a six-month period, consumed only 500 to 600 calories of relatively high-protein foods. They lost abdominal fat and displayed improved insulin sensitivity and reduced blood pressure.[10] The diet had a limited effect on glucose levels for overweight patients, however, indicating that longer treatment periods may be necessary for diabetes patients.[11] The advantage of this diet is that it requires minimal medical supervision. The disadvantage is that most obese and diabetes patients may find it difficult to remain on this diet for years, since it requires severe dietary restriction for two days every week. Further studies will be necessary to determine what the effects will be on diabetes patients.

A concern yet to be addressed is that alternating between a 2,000-calorie diet and a 500-calorie diet could trigger metabolic and sleep disorders resembling jet lag. Nonetheless, the 5:2 diet has been tried by thousands of people, particularly to lose weight, and many report a range of positive effects while being on it. Doctors should decide with their patients whether it may be incorporated into diabetes prevention or treatment therapies, preferably in combination with standard of care or as part of clinical trials.

FMD AND DIABETES TREATMENT

Diabetes drugs will interfere with or activate enzymes that can lower blood-glucose levels, but they will not target the multiple root causes for diabetes—some of which are understood and some of which are still emerging. The results of our one-hundred-patient randomized clinical trial are very promising: they show that undergoing three monthly cycles of the five-day FMD formulated to mimic fasting (750 to 1,100 calories per day) will lower many of the major risk factors for diabetes and metabolic syndrome, which increases the risk for heart disease, diabetes, and stroke.

METABOLIC REPROGRAMMING AND REGENERATION TO TREAT DIABETES

Scientists are wary of the word "cure" because it sounds like an exaggeration. However, for some patients with type 2 diabetes and the great majority of prediabetic patients, the combination of the dietary interventions described above could lead to a cure. I'm not saying everyone would be cured or that it's easy for diabetes patients to execute this plan. But the mouse and human data indicate that some and potentially many patients who follow the chronic dietary changes outlined in the first part of this chapter, or the periodic FMD, and preferably both, could eventually be free of type 2 diabetes, the most common type, especially if the treatment is started right after the initial diagnosis, when the pancreas is still functioning well. Note, as described below, that the combination of diabetes drugs and fasting or fasting-mimicking diets is

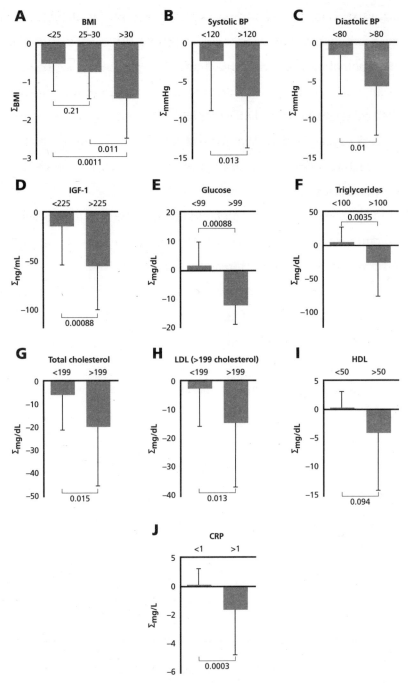

8.3. Changes in risk factors for diabetes and metabolic syndrome and other diseases from a 100-subject randomized clinical trial testing three monthly cycles of the FMD. The figure reports effects in both low-risk (left) and high-risk (right) participants.

dangerous and should be done as part of a clinical trial. Note also that although all the data, including clinical data, underline the high potential of these dietary changes in effectively treating diabetes, this will have to be demonstrated in a large randomized clinical trial and approved by the FDA before it can be prescribed to patients as a replacement for standard-of-care drugs for diabetes treatment. However, dietary interventions can serve as support to FDA approved therapies.

However, if you are at high risk for or suffer from diabetes, I encourage you to talk to your doctor and consider changing your everyday diet now, both for diabetes prevention and treatment. Our studies in mice and humans indicate that the FMD can prevent or potentially reverse diabetes by doing the following:

1. **Reducing abdominal and liver fat.** FMD pushes the body into a high fat-burning mode, mainly using abdominal/

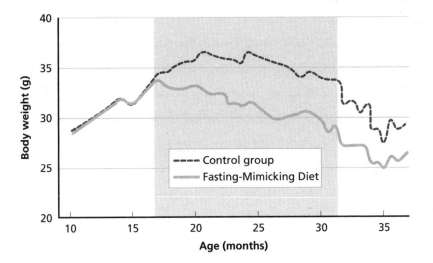

8.4. *Mice exposed to a fasting-mimicking diet lose weight while eating the same per month*

visceral fat but also liver fat, which are central to the promotion of diabetes and other diseases. Mice that undergo two cycles of the FMD a month, while eating the same total calories per month as mice on the regular diet, continue to lose weight, which suggests the fat-burning mode continues even after resuming a normal diet (see fig. 8.4).

2. **Promoting fat loss without muscle loss.** In the human clinical trial, obese participants lost approximately 9 pounds after three cycles of the FMD, and overweight participants lost an average of 4.5 pounds. However, the loss of lean body mass was either not observed or very small.

3. **Cell renewal/regeneration and autophagy.** By causing many damaged and old cells in different systems to die or reset, FMD flushes out bad cells and spurs regeneration inside the cell (autophagy) as well as new cell production through stem cell activation. This leads to regeneration and rejuvenation. In mice, we have demonstrated this process occurring in multiple systems, including the blood, the brain, the muscle, the liver, and the pancreas. In humans, data from clinical trials suggest the same regenerative process is occurring. Healthy subjects with low blood glucose or low blood pressure experienced little or no change after FMD cycles, protecting them from levels sinking dangerously low. However, the effects of FMD on glucose, blood pressure, and other risk factors for diabetes were much stronger in people who already had evidence of risk factors for aging and diseases at the beginning of the study (see fig. 8.3). These effects in humans, together with the data from mice, indicate either a rejuvenation or a regeneration of the damaged cells, or both.

**Fasting-Mimicking Diet cycles promote regeneration
and reverse pancreatic damage and diabetes**

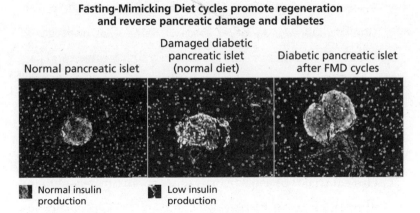

Normal pancreatic islet

Damaged diabetic
pancreatic islet
(normal diet)

Diabetic pancreatic islet
after FMD cycles

Normal insulin
production

Low insulin
production

*8.5. FMD cycles promote pancreatic regeneration to restore insulin
production and reverse both type 1 and type 2 diabetes in mice*

If muscle cells that respond poorly to insulin are either re-paired, rejuvenated, or regenerated, they can return to their normal function. (Not surprisingly, insulin resistance is relatively rare in young people, particularly in the non-obese, but is very common in older people, even if they are not obese.)

FMD, PANCREATIC REGENERATION, AND REVERSAL OF TYPE 1 AND TYPE 2 DIABETES IN MICE

In a recent paper, we showed that cycles of the FMD, in addition to improving the function of insulin, could promote the regeneration of insulin-producing beta cells and the reversal of both type 1 and type 2 diabetes symptoms in mice in which the pancreas could not generate sufficient insulin, resulting in very high glucose levels.[12] Remarkably, the FMD caused the activation of many pancreatic genes normally activated during embryonic/fetal development, suggesting that it can trigger a natural and highly coordinated regenerative response able to result in new and functioning beta cells, which can make normal levels of insulin.

A note about insulin and water-only fasting or similar: While death in people undergoing a prolonged fasting period is rare, when it did occur, it was in several cases associated with insulin use. A few patients have died by combining fasting with an insulin injection, probably because insulin normally works poorly in diabetes patients, and fasting partially reverses this effect. The same insulin injection that normally decreases glucose to healthy levels in a diabetic patient can cause a much more precipitous drop in a diabetic patient who is fasting—resulting in hypoglycemic shock and, in some cases, death. Similar albeit reduced dangers apply to the use of the fasting-mimicking diet.

A CAUTIONARY TALE (WITH A HAPPY ENDING)

I want to share an email I received from a stranger. It reinforces how powerful the periodic FMD and the daily Longevity Diet can be in preventing and treating disease, but it also demonstrates the dangers of self-treatment. This diabetic patient risked his life by combining insulin-like drugs with his own version of my Longevity Diet, and doing so without consulting his doctor.

Dear Dr. Longo,

You don't know it, but you saved my life. In December, I started my descent to hell with a paralysis of my left leg. By the night of Christmas I was in the hospital. A series of endless blood exams did not identify anything alarming but strong acid reflux, bad digestion, and continuous vomiting.

The gastroscopy, allergy, and food-intolerance tests did not show anything. According to the doctors, I was fine. I had eliminated meat, milk, and lactose-containing food from my diet since March, and I obtained some results. But I could not walk for more than 500 feet without gasping. My weight increased to 270 pounds without overeating, accompanied by an obvious edema in the legs and throughout the body; the imaging tests revealed a severe hepatic steatosis, which was turning into hepatic cirrhosis. My liver occupied a lot of my abdominal cavity, resulting in pressure to my stomach, which may have caused the reflux and a pleuritis in the lower part of the lung and continuous coughing.

On June 5, everything changed. I picked up a magazine and on its cover is the article about you: "Healing by Eating Less." I read the article and I was shocked. Keep in mind that I'm a diabetic person (insulin, NovoRapid 18 units 3 times per day, 22 units of Lantus at night—metformin pills and blood pressure medications). I adopted the diet described by you at the end of June, and everything changed. The results: 230 pounds, I walk/run for 3 miles per day and I'm taking a diving class. I eliminated the night diabetes drugs (Lantus) because it caused severe hypoglycemia at night, and reduced NovoRapid to 6 units in the morning, 10 units at lunch, and 8 units at dinner. I no longer take metformin. I eliminated all types of meats, milk, and lactose-containing foods, butter, margarine, fried food, alcohol, sweets, and sugars, and usually my glucose level does not go above 145. My doctors did not believe how well I was doing and wanted a copy of the article.

Fortunately, the patient did not adopt the FMD, only the Longevity Diet. But that was enough to resensitize his cells to insulin and cause severe hypoglycemia at night. He risked his life by making such a drastic change without consulting a doctor experienced in diet and diabetes to advise him during the transition. Had he also adopted the FMD, the combination of that and his diabetes drugs could have killed him.

The results of my research may have proven beneficial for this patient, but if you are diabetic I strongly discourage his self-administered approach. The big mistake, of course, was combining the diet with insulin. With just one visit to the right doctor before adopting the same diet and perhaps a periodic FMD, he could have done even better without risking hypoglycemic shock.

If your doctor resists helping you treat or prevent diabetes with dietary interventions, you should insist. It the doctor still refuses, look for a medical doctor specialized in integrative medicine, or contact L-Nutra and ask for a specialized doctor in their network.

I am not suggesting that conventional therapies do not work. But I believe medical doctors should prioritize therapies aimed at curing the patient, not just those that slow down the progression of disease. Recently I launched a training program to educate biologists, nutritionists, and medical doctors on the Longevity Diet and FMD. I hope to establish a network of specialized professionals in many countries to oversee patients wishing to use the dietary strategies described in this book.

TREATING OBESITY

Most of my work is geared toward preventing or finding a cure for common diseases, in most cases by acting on the aging process, and therefore the repair, protection, and regeneration of cellular components, cells, and organs. Usually I focus on animal and clinical studies related to obesity, diabetes, cancer, heart disease, or Alzheimer's, working at major universities and the hospitals associated with them. But every day people write to me, particularly when they've come to a dead end with traditional medicine. In such cases, I collect data about the individual patient and extrapolate from current scientific findings to devise a plan of action, which I then share with the patient and his or her doctor. I want to share two extreme cases among these, involving obesity.

CASE 1

I received a letter from a woman who had decided to do her own FMD. She wrote, "I have now experienced 15 five-day cycles of FMD. In total, I have lost 40 pounds (from 251 pounds to 211 pounds, that's 2.5 pounds per cycle), although due to a lack of availability of the ProLon FMD for about 10 months, I have regained a total of 6 pounds. My blood pressure has decreased from approximately 130 over 80 to approximately 120 over 70. During the three- to four-week period between cycles, I have more energy and am able to work longer hours without losing concentration.

"I find that the diet is not what I would call 'fun,' in that I enjoy eating a varied international diet and would prefer that to the FMD. However, I find that the short (five-day) period is tolerable, in that I don't feel hungry. Moreover, after five days I am able to resume my 'normal' diet and enjoy eating what I want. To maintain weight loss, I try not to binge, but I have an occasional hamburger, a couple of frozen yogurts, and even a pastry between cycles, so it isn't a difficult or major sacrifice."

CASE 2

The second case involves an obese man I helped who had tried everything to lose weight but nothing worked. He started at an unhealthy 245 pounds with a 50-inch waist and a 38 percent body fat composition, which placed him at a very high risk for developing diabetes. He did three cycles of the FMD and his weight, blood pressure, C-reactive protein (CRP; a measure of inflammation), and blood glucose levels all improved. The improvements were not major, however, because between cycles he would return to a high-fat, high-sugar, and high-starch diet and gain most of the weight back. I told him that considering his high disease risk, he should undergo four back-to-back cycles of the FMD diet under medical supervision.

I knew that fasting clinics regularly place patients on a 200-calorie-per-day diet for four weeks with few problems, so three weeks on FMD, providing at least 750 calories per day, was reasonable if the patient were very careful and worked closely with me and his doctor.

This strategy resulted in a loss of 30 pounds, a lot of it abdominal fat, and a major gain in energy and well-being. One year later, he had maintained his body weight and reported that FMD had changed his eating habits.

Clearly this multiple (two or more) FMD-cycle approach should be considered only when periodic cycles fail. Multiple cycles like these must be done with the approval and close monitoring of a doctor, preferably one who specializes in prolonged fasting therapies. Several potential side effects can result from this approach if it is followed improperly or if the wrong foods are consumed. Those side effects include an excessive drop in blood pressure or blood glucose, and malnourishment (deficiencies in certain vitamins, minerals, or essential nutrients). FMD can also produce a number of potential drug interactions, making a prolonged approach dangerous to some—for example, people receiving insulin therapy. Another concern is related to combining this major weight loss with a major weight gain. Multiple studies have shown that cycles of major weight loss followed by major weight regain can increase cardiovascular disease in both normal subjects and those already suffering from heart disease.[13]

Based on the abovementioned studies, it is particularly important to avoid weight losses and regains, thus the patient must be committed to continuing the FMD once a month after undergoing multiple consecutive FMD cycles. Please note that ProLon or any other FMD is only a tool that doctors can use to help manage obesity. We are now working toward performing clinical trials as part of the FDA approval process, but it takes time. Until that day, the information in this chapter provides a solid basis for dietary interventions that may complement standard diabetes prevention and treatment.

Next, a look at our very promising early studies into the Longevity Diet and FMD's positive countereffects on cardiovascular disease.

Chapter 9

FMD, Nutrition, and Cardiovascular Disease Prevention and Treatment*

[For their review of this chapter, I thank Kurt Hong, MD, PhD, associate professor and director of the USC Center for Clinical Nutrition, Los Angeles, and Andreas Michalsen, head physician at the Experimental and Clinical Research Center, Charité–University Medicine Berlin. I also thank Rafael De Cabo, PhD, Senior Investigator, Translational Gerontology Branch, National Institute on Aging (NIA), Baltimore.]

ACCORDING TO THE AMERICAN HEART ASSOCIATION, cardiovascular disease (CVD)—a category that includes coronary heart disease, stroke, coronary heart failure, high blood pressure, and arterial disease—kills around 801,000 people in the United States every year. That's about one in three deaths. In addition, around

---

* The contents of this chapter must not be used in self-diagnosis or the self-administration of therapies. This information is intended for medical professionals following your disease.

92 million Americans are living with some form of cardiovascular disease or the aftereffects of a stroke. Costs related to treatment and lost productivity are projected at around $316 billion. Clearly the drugs and other interventions being prescribed have not been very effective, and therefore the everyday Longevity Diet and FMD have the potential to reduce CVD incidence and progression. When it comes to cardiovascular disease, two very long studies on monkeys, conducted over decades, as well as multiple human studies serve as evidence of the power of certain diets in combating this widespread problem. I begin with a brief explanation of what they show us and where we can go from here.

Preventing Cardiovascular Disease in Monkeys

With a DNA sequence that is 93 percent identical to ours, rhesus macaques are perhaps the most humanlike organism in which we can study how lifespan responds to dietary interventions. They have a maximum lifespan of approximately forty years, making it possible to study them over a long but manageable period of time, and they develop many of the same diseases we do—including diabetes, cancer, and cardiovascular disease. Two monumental studies, one at the University of Wisconsin and one at the US National Institute on Aging (NIA), have measured how restricting calories by approximately 30 percent for life affects longevity and disease in rhesus monkeys.

The Wisconsin study, headed by Dr. Richard Weindruch, which ran for more than twenty years, concluded that a calorie-restricted (CR) diet lowers monkey mortality rates to 26 percent, compared with a 63 percent death rate in the control group.[1]

Forty-two percent of the monkeys on the regular diet developed prediabetes or diabetes, but none of the CR animals were diagnosed with either. In addition, cardiovascular diseases were reduced by 50 percent in the CR animals.[2]

In contrast to the Wisconsin study, the NIA study, led by Rafael de Cabo, found no apparent difference in the cause of death between the control and CR groups. Both groups showed a similar distribution of cardiovascular disease, amyloidosis, neoplasia, and general health deterioration.[3]

The difference between these two decades-long studies on diet in monkeys underscores the importance of diet composition in addition to limiting calories. In the NIA study, the control group received a healthy diet in which proteins were derived mainly from plant-based sources, including wheat, corn, soybean, and alfalfa, plus fish. Protein provided 17.3 percent of total calorie intake, along with 5 percent fat, 5 percent fiber, and 3.9 percent sucrose, plus vitamins and minerals. Finally, the animals were fed only twice a day, and their portions were adjusted for the age and body weight of each individual monkey.

In the University of Wisconsin study, milk (lactalbumin) was the only source of protein. The diet contained 10 percent fat (primarily from corn oil), 5 percent cellulose, and 28.5 percent sucrose. Unlike those in the NIA study, the Wisconsin monkeys in the control group were allowed to eat as much as they wanted, to better represent the typical Western diet.

In other words, the NIA control-group monkeys were kept to a healthy weight on a diet with similarities to the Longevity Diet described in this book, whereas the Wisconsin monkeys in the control group were on an animal-protein-based, high-sugar diet and were allowed to gain some weight. It is not surprising, then, that calorie restriction in the Wisconsin study was highly protective against aging and diseases, because the CR monkeys were being compared with control monkeys eating an unhealthy diet. The NIA control group, in contrast, was eating such a healthy diet that restricting it by 30 percent did not noticeably affect aging or most diseases, underlining the importance of the everyday diet, and supporting my conclusion throughout the book that for people who maintain an ideal longevity diet, the periodic FMD could be limited to twice a year.

Diet and Prevention of Cardiovascular Disease

Now back to humans. In chapter 4, I described the ideal Longevity Diet (which takes into account the Wisconsin and NIA monkey studies). However, milder versions of this diet exist, and their beneficial effects have been investigated in many studies. One of the most studied diets that has been shown to have effects on aging and disease, including cardiovascular disease, is the Mediterranean diet in its strictest form. The science behind its efficacy is rooted mostly in one of the Five Pillars—epidemiology—since few clinical trials and molecular studies have been carried out. Data from studies of centenarians show that extreme longevity has little to do with the Mediterranean diet per se. It is instead associated with specific ingredients and how heavily they are featured in diets common to the Mediterranean, Okinawa, Loma Linda, and Costa Rica. In other words, the Mediterranean diet *appears* to be a very good choice, but if we keep in mind all the pillars, the Longevity Diet, which includes the periodic FMD outlined in chapters 4 and 6, has the potential to be much more beneficial. Those unable to strictly follow that diet could still benefit by adding some components typical of both the Longevity and the Mediterranean diets.

Differences Between the Optimal Mediterranean and the Longevity Diet:

	Mediterranean Diet	Longevity Diet
Olive oil	High	High
Legumes	High	High
Unrefined cereals	High	High
Fruits	High	Low until old age, then higher
Cheese	Moderate	Absent/very low
Yogurt	Moderate	Low until age 65–70, then moderate
Wine	Moderate	Moderate
Meat & meat products	Low	Absent/very low
Milk	Low	Absent/very low
Eggs	Low	Absent/very low until age 65–70, then moderate
Butter	Low	Absent/very low
Protein levels	Not addressed	Low until age 65–70, then moderate
General food consumption	Not addressed	Normal until age 65–70, then sufficient to maintain a healthy muscle mass
Time-restricted feeding	Not addressed	11–12 hr eating window central to plan

Many studies have shown that the Mediterranean diet described above is associated with reduced incidence of chronic diseases, including cardiovascular disease.[4] For example, a study at the University of Florence looked at data obtained from 4.1 million subjects and found a clear correlation between a lower risk for cardiovascular disease and a greater adherence to the Mediterranean diet.[5]

As with the Longevity Diet, consumption of olive oil and nuts is consistently associated with longevity and protection from cardiovascular disease. To understand whether olive oil and nuts in fact provide protection from diseases, a study at Spain's Barcelona University followed 7,447 men and women ages fifty-eight to eighty at risk for developing cardiovascular disease. These subjects consumed a Mediterranean diet supplemented with either one liter of extra-virgin olive oil per week or with 30 grams of mixed nuts (15 grams of walnuts, 7.5 grams of hazelnuts, 7.5 grams of almonds). Subjects in the control group instead consumed a reduced-fat diet.[6] The research team observed a reduction in cardiovascular events (stroke, heart attack, etc.) in both the Mediterranean diet group supplemented with olive oil and the one supplemented with nuts.[7] More than five years later, observation of the same group revealed that the intake of mono- and polyunsaturated fats, such as those contained in olive and other vegetable oils, was associated with reduced cardiovascular disease, but a diet rich in saturated and trans fats increased cardiovascular disease.[8] Notably, the intake of saturated fats from fish and plant-based sources (nuts, etc.) was associated with reduced cardiovascular disease and death.[9]

A Harvard study, discussed earlier, of nearly 130,000 men and women—which recorded more than 20,000 deaths, 5,204 of those from cardiovascular disease—showed that those in the group on a low-carbohydrate, mostly animal-based, high-protein diet were twice as likely to die of any cause, and had a 40 percent higher risk of dying of cardiovascular disease.[10] When the diet was vegetable-based but still low in carbohydrates, it was no longer associated with higher cardiovascular disease. In fact, it appeared to reduce diseases further.

Another study following a large group of middle-aged men indicated that high intake of proteins from animal-based sources increased the rates of stroke and ischemic heart disease, whereas a higher plant-based protein intake was protective.[11]

As we and others have shown, people with high vegetable-based protein intake normally have lower or much lower overall protein intake, suggesting that the lower incidence of disease may be caused by both the beneficial effects of plant-based food and the lower overall protein intake, compared with people eating high levels of animal-based proteins.

A study of 43,396 women in Sweden reported a 5 percent increase in the incidence of cardiovascular disease with each 5-gram increase in protein intake and 20-gram reduction in carbohydrate intake.[12]

Another study evaluating 2,210 cases of nonfatal infarcts and 952 deaths from heart disease also concluded that a high intake of red meat and fat correlates with an elevated risk of heart disease in women, whereas intake of nuts and beans reduces the risk.[13]

When my PhD adviser Roy Walford was in Biosphere 2, he and the other seven residents of the sealed environment in the Arizona desert were on a calorie-restricted diet for almost two years.[14] Their meals, providing fewer than 1,800 calories a day, were mostly vegetarian—consisting of fruits, grains, peas, beans, peanuts, greens, potatoes, plus other vegetables and small quantities of goat's milk and yogurt (about 84 grams per day), with very small quantities of goat meat, pork, fish, and eggs.[15] The eight Biospherians showed remarkable changes in risk factors for cardiovascular diseases after adopting this diet.

Several studies have confirmed the Biosphere 2 results and have also shown that calorie restriction reduces inflammation (CRP levels) and additional markers associated with cardiovascular diseases.[16]

Taken together, these studies confirm that many of the risk factors for heart disease and stroke can be prevented and even very effectively treated by very specific dietary interventions. However, as we saw with the rhesus monkey studies, prolonged calorie restriction is an extreme intervention that produces both benefits and problems.

Risk Factor	Beginning of experiment	During experiment (undergoing caloric restriction)
Blood pressure (mmHg)	108/77	90/58
Cholesterol (LDL) (mg/dL)	105	60
Triglycerides (mg/dL)	115	80
BMI	23	19
Fasting blood glucose (mg/dL)	92	70

9.1. *How the Biosphere 2 experiment influenced risk factors for cardiovascular disease*

For example, as figure 9.1 shows, the body mass index after chronic calorie restriction typically reaches a value of 19, even for men. The average BMI of a Holocaust survivor was 14.2. Approaching an emaciated state can have a wide range of negative consequences on wound healing and the ability to fight infectious diseases.

We need to take advantage of what we learned from these powerful calorie-restriction studies and use this information to identify dietary and other effective interventions that don't lead to excessive weight loss and potentially severe side effects.

Diet and Treatment of Cardiovascular Disease

Several studies have investigated the role of dietary intervention in the treatment of cardiovascular diseases. In one randomized study from the 1990s, people were placed on the "Ornish diet," named for UC San Francisco medical researcher Dean Ornish. The diet consists of no animal products, no caffeine, 10 percent of calories from fat obtained from grains, vegetables, fruit, beans, legumes, or soy foods, and only 12 grams of sugar per day. Together with mild to moderate exercise and stress management, study participants saw their risk of developing coronary athero-sclerosis improve after just one year.[17] Twenty-three of the twenty-eight patients on this diet showed regression of atherosclerosis; meanwhile, the health of the subjects on the control diet declined.[18]

After five years on the Ornish diet, the study group's positron emission tomography (PET) scans showed abnormalities associated with heart disease had decreased, compared with the control group's scans, in measurements taken both at rest and under drug-induced heart stress.[19]

A similar diet, tested first in a small group and eventually monitored in a larger group of patients diagnosed with cardiovascular disease, was designed by Cleveland Clinic surgeon Caldwell Esselstyn. Similar to the Ornish diet, Esselstyn's regimen contains no meat, poultry, fish, dairy, oil of any kind, nuts, or avocado. It allows vegetables, legumes, whole grains, and fruits.

The focus of the Esselstyn diet is to maintain cholesterol at very low levels. In the original study, he placed twenty-four patients with severe coronary artery disease on the diet and followed them for twelve years. In all eighteen patients who stayed on the diet, coronary heart disease was either arrested or regressed. After twelve years, seventeen of the eighteen patients maintained a cholesterol level of 145 mg/dL.

However, there are several limitations to the Esselstyn and Ornish diets. First, because they are so restrictive, the chance of long-term compliance in the general population is uncertain at best. Second, both diets overlook the benefits of nuts, other plant-based fats, and fish. These foods have been associated with decreased, not increased, heart disease.[20] The consumption of fish, olive oil, and nuts in some combination is common among record-longevity populations, including the Seventh-day Adventists of Loma Linda (although most don't eat fish), the Greeks of Ikaria, the Italians of Calabria and Sardinia, and the Japanese in Okinawa (although they don't consume high levels of olive oil).

Support for the inclusion of these foods extends beyond epidemiological, clinical, and centenarian studies. Calorie-restriction studies in humans have not prohibited nuts, olive oil, other fats, or fish, yet they have reported major decreases in total cholesterol. CR study subjects reached 125 mg/dL and 60 low-density lipoprotein (LDL) mg/dL levels, both far lower than the 150 (total) and 80 (LDL) mg/dL that Esselstyn considers healthy levels providing high protection against diseases.

In summary, although the Esselstyn and Ornish diets appear to be effective in the treatment of cardiovascular disease, I recommend talking to your cardiologist about adopting the cardiovascular diseases treatment diet outlined at the end of this chapter, which takes into account their studies together with the Five Pillars of Longevity. My modifications allow the reintroduction of relatively high levels of nuts, olive oil, and certain fish containing high levels of omega-3 fatty acids, such as salmon. I also reduce the consumption of fruit, pasta, bread, and daily proteins, which my research team and others have associated with a high risk of age-related diseases.

Periodic Fasting-Mimicking Diets in the Prevention and Treatment of Cardiovascular Disease

My laboratory has focused on interventions that are simple and effective, and that minimize changes people don't want to make. Our approach with cardiovascular diseases is not based on blocking the activity of enzymes, such as those that produce cholesterol or affect blood pressure. Rather, our goal is to switch *on* the body's ability to promote cellular protection, regeneration, and rejuvenation, leading to improved function and a return to a more youthful, healthy state.

As with cancer and diabetes, the effects of the periodic FMD on risk factors for cardiovascular diseases are impressive, although they need to be confirmed by larger clinical studies.[21] When we tested the FMD in humans, subjects displayed lower cardiovascular disease and inflammation markers after three diet cycles, without any adverse effects. Other findings included reduced body weight and body fat without loss of lean mass.[22] Three cycles of the FMD performed once a month for five days, followed by a return to a normal diet, reduced abdominal circumference in all participants by 1.6 inches.

However, in general, FMD cycles were far more effective in individuals with high levels of risk factors for cardiovascular diseases than they were in healthy individuals. For example, systolic blood pressure dropped about 7 mmHg in subjects with moderately high blood pressure; triglycerides fell by 25 mg/dL in subjects with high triglycerides; and bad cholesterol (LDL) went down by nearly 22 mg/dL among at-risk individuals. Notably, three cycles of the FMD returned the levels of CRP, an important inflammatory risk factor for cardiovascular disease, to the normal range in the great majority of study subjects (figure 9.2).

Summary of the FMD
and Cardiovascular Disease,
Results of Clinical Trials,
Prevention, and Treatment

In our human clinical study involving one hundred subjects, FMD cycles affected many of the major risk factors or markers contributing to or associated with cardiovascular diseases, particularly in individuals at high risk. The results of the FMD related to cardiovascular diseases include the following:

1. Reduced abdominal fat and circumference
2. Major drop in the inflammatory risk factor, C-reactive protein
3. Reduction in total and LDL cholesterol
4. Lowering of triglycerides
5. Reduction in systolic and diastolic blood pressure
6. Reduction in fasting glucose

The following are my guidelines for the prevention and treatment of cardiovascular disease:

PREVENTION

1. Follow the Longevity Diet (chapter 4) and the exercise guidelines (chapter 5).
2. Undergo periodic fasting-mimicking diets. For very healthy individuals with no cardiovascular-disease risk factors, we recommend FMD once every six months. For those over-

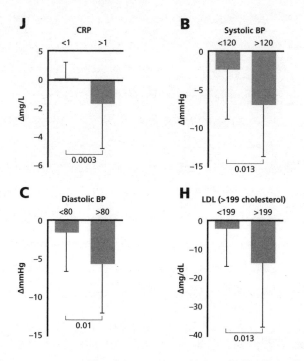

9.2. C-reactive protein, blood pressure, and LDL cholesterol, all risk factors for cardiovascular disease, decrease after three cycles of the FMD

weight with multiple risk factors for cardiovascular diseases, including a family history of heart disease or stroke, we recommend FMD once a month until normal weight is achieved, then it can be reduced according to the guidelines in chapter 6.

TREATMENT

The best and safest strategy is to talk to your cardiologist about taking components of the Esselstyn, Ornish, Walford, and Longevity diets and combining them with new information emerging from clinical and epidemiological studies discussed in this chapter. For more specifics on all the below guidelines, see chapter 4.

- No: red meat, poultry, or other meats (excluding fish)
- No: dairy
- Yes: fish
- Yes: large amounts of vegetables (best if organic)
- Yes: legumes, including beans, lentils, garbanzo beans, peas (best if organic)
- Yes: whole grains, including pasta and bread, but less than 100 grams per day
- Yes: fruits, but only one or two a day (e.g., one apple or orange, two handfuls of blueberries, blackberries, or strawberries)
- Yes: olive oil (about 80 grams per day)
- Yes: nuts (about 30 grams a day of walnuts, almonds, or hazelnuts)
- Limit all eating to eleven to twelve hours a day (e.g., between 8 a.m. and 7 or 8 p.m. only).
- Limit meals to twice a day plus a low-sugar, high-fiber snack with fewer than 100 calories, if you are above BMI 25.
- Limit sugar to less than 10 grams per day.
- Eat approximately 0.31 to 0.36 grams of protein per pound of body weight per day. If you weigh 130 pounds, that comes to about 40 to 47 grams of protein per day, of which 30 grams should be consumed in a single meal to maximize muscle synthesis.
- Exercise as directed in chapter 5.
- The diet I propose differs from the Ornish diet in that it allows high levels of fat from fish, olive oil, and nuts. However, it does not go as far as the Barcelona study's diet fat allowance, which permits close to one liter of olive oil per week. Because the Barcelona study diet clearly protects against cardiovascular

disease, the diet presented here is a compromise that factors in decades of work and evidence produced by Ornish, Esselstyn, and others indicating that very low-fat intake may be preferable while also considering more recent studies suggesting that there is little evidence that a decreased consumption of olive oil and nuts will produce a beneficial effect.

- Talk to your doctor about using the dietary treatments described here as an integrative strategy.
- Undergo periodic FMD. Remind your doctor that hypertension medications should not be taken with FMD unless it is clear that your blood pressure will remain within the normal range.

Remember, because the dietary interventions described in this chapter have not yet been tested in large randomized clinical trials for the treatment of cardiovascular disease, they should be used only in support of standard of care. Our early results are certainly promising enough that you and your doctor should bear them in mind as we continue to work toward larger trials and FDA approval. The same goes for the next area we will look at, neurodegenerative diseases, especially Alzheimer's and other dementias.

Chapter 10

FMD and Nutrition in the Prevention and Treatment of Alzheimer's and Other Neurodegenerative Diseases[*]

[For their review of this chapter, I thank neurologist Markus Bock, a specialist in the application of the ketogenic diet and fasting-mimicking diet at the Experimental and Clinical Research Center, Charité–University Medicine Berlin, and Patrizio Odetti, chief of geriatrics at the University of Genova San Martino Hospital.]

BRAIN FUNCTION AND DAMAGE HAS LONG been a scholarly focus and passion of mine. As with aging, it represents a daunting scientific challenge. The brain is commonly afflicted by diseases, including Alzheimer's and Parkinson's, that are devastating to sufferers and those around them. Yet I know and have spent time with many very elderly people who remain sharp and witty into

---

[*] The contents of this chapter must not be used in self-diagnosis or the self-administration of therapies. This information is intended for medical professionals following your disease.

their nineties and hundreds. My goal is to help as many people as possible live to a very old age with normal mental faculties. This chapter focuses mostly on Alzheimer's disease and other dementias—specifically how nutrition and an FMD may affect their incidence and progression. Although Parkinson's disease is also one of my research group's areas of interest, we have not yet completed studies related to it. We have high hopes that the Longevity Diet and FMD will have beneficial effects on Parkinson's, but it would be premature to speculate on possible outcomes before performing basic and clinical research on this disease.

Alzheimer's Disease

Alzheimer's disease (AD) accounts for 60 to 80 percent of all dementias. It is characterized by a loss of memory that interferes with normal daily tasks. In the early stages of the disease, patients have difficulty remembering newly acquired information. Later they become disoriented, show changes in mood and behavior, and often grow suspicious of family members or caregivers, whom they fail to recognize and remember. As the memory loss becomes severe, patients may have difficulty speaking, walking, and even swallowing.

When I first started working on AD in the laboratory of USC neurobiologist Caleb Finch in 1997, the great promise in combatting the disease was a vaccine against a protein called beta-amyloid, which accumulates in the brains of AD patients and which scientists generally agree is somehow involved in the disease, since it is linked to both the hereditary and nonhereditary forms. Twenty years later, this strategy has yet to produce any effective treatment, and hundreds of laboratories are still searching for a cure. It is also no longer clear that beta-amyloid accumulation has a primary causal role in the disease.

While we continue to search for a cure though, even a five-year delay in the average age of Alzheimer's disease diagnosis would cut the number of patients by nearly half, since onset occurs at such an advanced age that many patients would die of another cause before developing the disease. Thus, AD is an excellent candidate for the use of dietary interventions such as the FMD, with wide effects on the aging process, which could delay AD onset or progression.

Prevention of Alzheimer's Disease in Mice

Not surprisingly, the major risk factor for AD is aging. Incidence of the disease increases by more than a hundredfold from age sixty to age ninety-five. Mouse studies have provided a platform for understanding Alzheimer's disease, since the human genes known to cause AD can be introduced into the mouse genome, promoting some of the memory loss and learning deficits observed in Alzheimer's patients.

Again, it is sad that we must sacrifice mice to identify interventions for Alzheimer's. But before we can begin human testing, we have no choice but to do preliminary tests in mice. It's worth noting that the mice used in our AD studies do not appear to suffer; the cognitive decline caused by the mutations we introduce is similar to what occurs in humans with AD who reach very old age.

Thanks to these studies in mice, my group is now ready to start a clinical trial on the use of FMD in the prevention and treatment of AD together with a group of clinical geriatricians and neurologists at the University of Genova. We have already performed preliminary studies on the effects of the FMD on cognitive performance in normal participants and obtained positive and very promising results, which serve as a strong foundation for the Alzheimer studies. The point of this section is not to review all mouse studies related to diet and Alzheimer's. Rather, the goal is to lay the foundation for specific diets in the prevention and treatment of neurodegenerative diseases.

Our first study attempted to delay the onset of Alzheimer's disease by regulating the genes that accelerate aging. We used "triple transgenic" mice, which have three of the mutated human genes associated with Alzheimer's disease (APP, PS1, and tau). Because AD in the great majority of cases occurs after age seventy, we opted against using a chronic low-calorie diet, since even if it proved effective, it could not be safely adopted by elderly people. We decided to regulate the activity of the two major sets of genes accelerating aging by tricking the cells, giving the mice a normal diet that lacked the nine essential amino acids (those the body cannot generate: isoleucine, leucine, lysine, methionine, phenylalanine, threonine, tryptophan, valine, and arginine). We also gave the mice excess quantities of the nonessential amino acids, which the human body can make and therefore does not need to obtain from the diet. In other words, the test diet was identical to the normal diet but contained fewer essential amino acids and more nonessential amino acids.

Starting at young to middle age, the mice received this diet every other week, alternating with a normal diet. The potent effect of this minimal change is obvious from the 75 percent reduction we detected in the levels of the pro-aging and cancer growth factor IGF-1 in the mice while on the diet. Notably, the effect of this dietary intervention on IGF-1 levels continued even after the mice returned to their normal diet. Months later, the mice placed on the protein-restricted diet every other week had better performance in several different cognitive tests, indicating that they were protected from Alzheimer's disease symptoms.

These results are evidence of the potential of nutritechnology—that is, understanding the effect of food composition on specific genes and pathways in the quest for therapeutic diets that are minimally disruptive yet have effects comparable or superior to drug therapy. This is different from the concept of "nutraceuticals," which in most cases are foods engineered for concentrated levels of particular molecules that have specific biological or med-

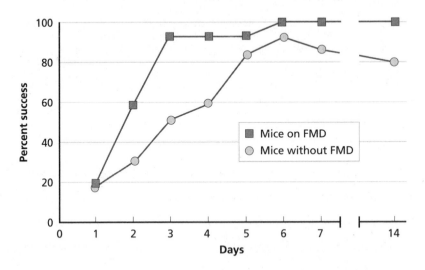

10.1. *Improvement of cognitive tests in mice exposed to fasting-mimicking diet cycles*

ical functions. For example, concentrated vitamin C obtained from acerola can be considered a nutraceutical.

In a study I have already mentioned, mice received a reduced-calorie FMD for four-day cycles twice a month (eight days a month total), starting in middle age. In old age, these mice learned and remembered much better than mice in the control group (see fig. 10.1). We observed performance improvements in all tests, including motor coordination (on a rotating wheel), and both long-term and short-term memory.

The FMD cycles had profound effects on genes that play key roles in the aging process, including aging of the brain. Researchers at the US National Institute on Aging have performed many studies in this area, focusing on alternate-day fasting. Receiving no food one day and a normal diet the next day, these mice consistently showed improvements in learning and memory function. The benefits applied to both normal mice and mice with Alzheimer's disease.[1]

We are now ready to begin clinical trials to test the effect of similar but less calorie-restricted diets in humans.

Dietary Prevention of Alzheimer's Disease in Humans

The periodic FMD, because it promotes a longer and generally healthier lifespan, is recommended for most people, but because it provides a very low level of calories, it is not recommended for people over the age of seventy. What would be the point of adopting a diet that prevents Alzheimer's disease if the same diet promoted a deficiency in the immune system or made the patient frail? Thus, before a dietary intervention can be recommended, it is imperative that its potential to prevent or treat a disease or condition outweighs its potential to cause adverse side effects. Thus, the minimal risks of using an FMD in a sixty-five-year-old would be justified if this person was at high risk for developing Alzheimer's; this should be considered only until age seventy, or possibly older depending on the ability to maintain a normal weight and muscle mass, and based on the individual's overall health status and the opinion of a neurologist. Notably, several studies indicate that a calorie-restricted diet improves and prevents loss of muscle mass in older animals and therefore further studies are needed to determine whether periodic FMDs would have positive or negative effects on muscle mass and strength in the elderly. With the availability of inexpensive and highly specific DNA testing, we can now also consider diets tailored for the prevention of a specific disease in individuals. For example, the APOE protein, responsible for carrying cholesterol and cholesterol-like molecules, comes in three forms: APOE2, APOE3, and APOE4. For people—particularly women—who have two copies of the APOE4 gene, the risk of developing Alzheimer's disease is fifteen times higher than average. In the general population, the chance of having AD after age eighty-five is more than 40 percent; for someone with two copies (alleles) of the APOE4 gene, the risk shoots up to 91 percent—with half of them developing the disease by age sixty-eight.[2] I encourage anyone whose parents or grandparents had Alzheimer's disease to pursue genetic testing to determine if they have risk factors for the disease. If the tests come back positive, they may want to talk to their doctor about adopting the dietary recommendations that follow.

The Longevity Diet
Plus Excess Olive Oil and Nuts

The periodic FMD may be effective in cognitive disease prevention in mice and possibly humans, but everyday diet also plays a central role in cognitive health. Although we are still conducting our studies into the positive effects of the Longevity Diet on neurodegenerative diseases, an everyday diet that *has* been shown to be protective against cognitive decline is the Mediterranean diet in combination with high levels of olive oil.[3]

A six-year study in Barcelona, Spain, originally designed as a cardiovascular study (and mentioned in the last chapter) monitored 447 volunteers (with a mean age of sixty-seven years) who were at high cardiovascular risk but cognitively healthy. Participants were randomly assigned to a Mediterranean diet supplemented with either extra virgin olive oil or 30 grams of nuts per day, or a control diet in which they were advised to reduce dietary fat. Participants on the Mediterranean diet plus olive oil or nuts performed better in cognitive testing than those on the low-fat control diet.[4]

In people over age sixty—and likely also in younger people—a Mediterranean diet supplemented with either olive oil or nuts is associated with improved cognitive function. However, an analysis of many studies on the Mediterranean diet and neurodegenerative diseases concluded that adherence to the Mediterranean diet only decreases the risk of neurodegenerative diseases by 13 percent.[5] Thus, in order to optimize brain health and delay or prevent Alzheimer's onset, I recommend the Longevity Diet plus additional nutrients including olive oil and nuts, as described below. Though the efficacy of this diet in the prevention of dementia has not been demonstrated yet, it has a higher potential for significant impact since it represents a stricter version of the Mediterranean diet and includes many additional nutrients of reported benefit.

Coffee and Coconut Oil

The role of coffee in health and longevity has been controversial. Although earlier studies included coffee as a risk factor for a variety of age-related diseases, including cancer and heart disease, later more careful studies indicate that moderate coffee consumption may in fact protect against diseases, including Parkinson's, type 2 diabetes, and liver disease. A few studies suggest that coffee may also protect against Alzheimer's.

Researchers at the University of South Carolina reviewed studies published between 1966 and 2014 assessing the relationship between coffee consumption and dementias. They examined eleven studies of a total of 29,000 participants. Overall, coffee drinkers and non–coffee drinkers showed no difference in their risk of developing dementia. However, the group with the highest coffee consumption had an approximately 30 percent reduction in the risk of developing Alzheimer's disease. It is possible that drinking three or four cups of coffee a day may protect against Alzheimer's, as it was shown to protect against Parkinson's.[6] This may be caused in part by coffee's high polyphenol content. However, this type of coffee consumption could cause side effects, and its use should be considered only if you are at high risk for AD, and then under medical supervision.

Coconut oil contains high levels of saturated fat. But unlike other dietary saturated fats, which are composed mainly of long-chain fatty acids (fats with 13 to 21 carbons in the chain), coconut oil contains a high level of medium-chain fatty acids (MCFA, or fats with 6 to 12 carbons in the chain). MCFA are easily converted into ketone bodies, the same molecules produced at high levels during fasting. The brain begins to utilize ketones as a major source of energy during prolonged fasting periods and when glucose is scarce.

In a study of patients with Alzheimer's disease, consumption of 40 milliliters (1.5 fluid ounces) per day of extra virgin coconut oil resulted in an improvement in cognitive status. This finding is consistent with other studies suggesting medium-chain fatty acids protect against dementia. While coconut oil's protective role must be confirmed in large clinical studies, the published data indicates it may improve cognition in Alzheimer's disease patients.[7] Notably, the American Heart Association includes coconut oil among the potentially harmful foods containing saturated fats. Whether this concern is appropriate is hotly debated, but the possibility that regular use of coconut oil could increase cardiovascular disease should be considered when using it to prevent or treat dementias.

"Bad" Fats and Alzheimer's Disease

While the medium-length fats in coconut oil and the mono-unsaturated fats in olive oil may protect against Alzheimer's disease, the opposite is true of saturated and other fats, the "bad" fats, which may increase the risk of developing dementia in addition to cardiovascular disease. Several studies indicate that consuming high levels of saturated or trans fatty acids increases the risk of dementia. In studies conducted at the Chicago Health and Aging Project, consumption of saturated and trans fatty acids was associated with an increased risk of AD.[8] These findings support adoption of the Longevity Diet, which is nearly free of the saturated fats and trans fats found in high quantities in animal-derived foods (especially red meat, butter, cheese, whole milk, pork, and candy).[9]

Sufficient Nourishment

Certain vitamins and other nutrients have been proposed to be neuroprotective—that is, capable of protecting neurons against damage. This view is probably simplistic, but some studies have implicated deficiencies in omega-3 fatty acids, B vitamins, and vitamins C, D, and E in brain aging and dementias. To date, most have failed to show a clear association between high-dose supplementation of these vitamins and nutrients and protection against dementias.

That said, every diet should contain a sufficient level of foods rich in all these nutrients (see appendix B for foods containing the highest levels of these nutrients). In fact, a review of studies indicates that AD patients have lower levels of folate and vitamins A, B12, C, and E. It would not be surprising if, in the future, certain deficiencies were found to contribute to AD. So while supplementing with high levels of vitamins or fatty acids may not be proven as protective, it avoids the risk of developing a deficiency, which could accelerate brain degeneration and dementias. Foods rich in vitamins may reduce the risk of AD but, for example, B vitamin supplementation was found to be largely ineffective, except in countries where food is not fortified with the folate vitamin.[10]

Age-Appropriate Weight and Abdominal Circumference

The association between body mass index (which takes into account a person's weight relative to height) and cognition is complex and varies according to age. In younger and middle-age adults, a high BMI is associated with reduced cognition or a higher risk of dementia once these adults reach old age. However, a slightly higher BMI in older adults is associated with improved cognition and lower mortality. Thus, it is important to maintain a healthy weight and ideal abdominal circumference up to age sixty-five; beyond that point, the goal should be to reach the upper limit of the healthy BMI and abdominal circumference ranges. For men, a BMI in the 22 to 23 range may be ideal up to age sixty-five to seventy-five, but beyond that age, a BMI in the 23 to 25 range may be preferable in order to avoid loss of muscle mass and other detrimental deficiencies.

This goal could be achieved by adding small amounts of foods not permitted or very restricted under the Longevity Diet, such as eggs, goat's or sheep's cheese and yogurt, dark chocolate, fruit, and higher levels of fish and seafood. These foods should be consumed only in moderation even at older ages. Adding them to the Longevity Diet may help prevent weight loss and muscle loss, especially when protein consumption (0.4 grams of protein per pound of body weight) is combined with muscle training and exercise (see chapter 5).[11]

Dietary Treatment of Alzheimer's Disease

Dietary interventions to prevent dementias—including coconut oil, olive oil, and the Longevity Diet—may also help patients with Alzheimer's disease or a condition called mild cognitive impairment, which often precedes dementia.

Unlike their role in treating cancer, diabetes, and cardiovascular disease, however, the role of dietary interventions in the treatment of Alzheimer's disease and other dementias is little understood and still speculative. Because AD is devastating to patients and their families, and because most AD patients cannot afford to wait for future studies, I will describe the mouse studies we have completed and the studies we are about to perform in AD patients, which I believe have potential.

Again, the purpose of these interventions isn't necessarily to cure AD but to try to delay its onset by five or ten years or more. Only a neurologist specialized in AD can determine whether any individual patient should try the diet. It must be understood that this is an unproven and risky strategy, which needs clinical testing in large trials before its safety and efficacy can be established. It would be best to try the following recommendations as part of an approved clinical trial.

As I mentioned, we had positive results in a mouse study alternating weeklong cycles of a protein-free diet supplemented with nonessential amino acids and weeklong cycles of a normal high-protein diet. With the input of an experienced neurologist, AD patients could try weekly cycles of a low-protein diet (0.1 to 0.15 grams of protein per pound of body weight) alternating with a relatively high-protein diet (0.45 grams of protein per pound of body weight). The patient would eat a diet based on carbohydrates and "good" fats (no meat, fish, eggs, milk, or cheese and low levels of legumes) for one week, followed by a normal and high-nourishment Longevity Diet the next week. The diet should include daily supplements of coconut oil (40 milliliters). During the "nourishment week," salmon and other fish high in omega-3 oils (see appendix B) should be eaten at least three times a week, with care taken to avoid high-mercury fish.

Continue these week-on, week-off cycles of very low protein and normal protein for at least six months to see if (1) cognitive performance improves and (2) the patient maintains normal weight and muscle mass and does not develop other symptoms. If the patient loses more than 5 percent of body weight or muscle mass, further cycles of the diet should be delayed until the patient returns to a healthy weight.

Another admittedly risky option is to use the monthly FMD, which we have tested in people ages twenty to seventy but not in older subjects or in AD patients (see chapter 6). In a small and preliminary study, we observed improvements in cognitive performance in subjects who received three cycles of the monthly FMD. This is consistent with the strong effects of the twice-a-month FMD started in middle age on neural regeneration and the improved cognitive performance in mice once they reach old age.[12]

Note that FMD is potentially very risky in elderly subjects, especially those who are frail, are low-weight, or have lost weight during the progression of the disease. In the periods between FMD cycles, patients should follow a high-nourishment, plant- and fish-based diet that's relatively high in protein (0.45 gram of protein per pound of body weight).

I emphasize once more that these interventions should be considered only in the absence of other viable options and based on the recommendation of a specialized neurologist, with the precautions and warnings listed above and preferably as part of a clinical trial.

Exercise Both Body and Mind

Remaining both physically and mentally active has been shown to protect against age-related dementias. A review of all the studies on exercise and dementia, covering eight hundred patients and eighteen randomized clinical trials, concluded that physical activity—particularly aerobic exercise, such as running and swimming—improves cognitive function in patients with dementia (see the exercise guidelines in chapter 5).[13]

Exercise is important in both the prevention and treatment of dementias. Naturally, for frail and older patients, a stationary bicycle may be more appropriate than running or swimming. Pedal resistance can be adjusted to achieve the right level of difficulty to challenge but avoid physical harm to the patient.

Another way to ward off AD and other dementias is to maintain brain activity. Reading, solving puzzles, and playing computer games have all been shown to improve cognition and help prevent or delay dementias.[14]

Summary: Prevention and Treatment of Neurodegenerative Diseases

Prevention

The following are guidelines for people at high risk of developing dementias (given family history or early cognitive decline):

1. Adopt the Longevity Diet and the periodic FMD.
2. Incorporate plenty of olive oil (50 milliliters per day) and nuts (30 grams per day).
3. Drink coffee. For people at relatively low risk of AD, keep it to one or two cups a day; for people at high risk, drink up to three or four cups a day. Speak to your doctor if you have problems.
4. Take 40 milliliters of coconut oil per day but consider poten-

tial heart disease risk (people with or at risk for cardiovascular disease should not use coconut oil).

5. Avoid saturated fats and trans fats.

6. Avoid all animal-based products with the exception of low-mercury fish and cheese or other dairy products from goat's milk.

7. Follow a high-nourishment diet containing omega-3, B vitamins, and vitamins C, D, and E.

8. Take a multivitamin and mineral every day.

Treatment

The following are guidelines for people who have already been diagnosed with AD or dementia. This treatment plan must be approved and supervised by a neurologist and should be combined with standard of care.

1. Follow all the dementia-prevention dietary recommendations above.

2. Talk to your neurologist about following cycles of a protein- and essential amino acid–deficient diet followed by normal calorie intake and/or cycles of the periodic FMD.

   With AD and other diseases that are later in onset, it's important to remember that calorie- and nutrient-restricted diets are potentially dangerous to the elderly, so the neurologist on the case should work with a registered dietitian to optimize the effects on brain function while minimizing risks and side effects.

Although our studies into AD are perhaps the most speculative, this is an area I feel especially passionate about. By acting on the aging process using strategies like the Longevity Diet, it is possible to delay and even prevent diseases and remain as healthy as Emma Morano or Salvatore Caruso, who remembered well not only what they had done an hour earlier but also remembered many stories and even songs from their youth. This is my ambitious vision, and we're working with labs and researchers around the world to help make it possible.

FMD and Nutrition in the Prevention and Treatment of Inflammatory and Autoimmune Diseases*

[For their review of this chapter, I thank Kurt Hong, MD, PhD, associate professor and director of the USC Center for Clinical Nutrition, Los Angeles, and Andreas Michalsen, head physician, at the Experimental and Clinical Research Center, Charité–University Medicine Berlin.]

Aging and the Autoimmune System

As we age, we suffer damage to, or malfunction of, the cells of our immune system. White blood cells central to the immune system—including T cells, macrophages, and neutrophils—naturally produce inflammatory factors. These normally play a central role in coordinating many different healthy immune

---

* The contents of this chapter must not be used in self-diagnosis or the self-administration of therapies. This information is intended for medical professionals following your disease.

functions, ranging from combatting and killing bacteria and viruses to killing and disposing of damaged human cells, including cancer cells.

But as we get older, and also in association with disease, production of both immune cells and these inflammatory factors can become dysregulated. When this happens, inflammation can be activated even when it is not needed. This can result in a low-level systemic inflammation involving the entire body. In some cases, this inflammation is followed by the development of a strong immunity against normal cells or molecules within cells, resulting in a self-recognition, in which the immune system attacks parts of its own body—this is what occurs in autoimmune diseases such as multiple sclerosis, Crohn's, and type 1 diabetes.

One way to determine whether someone has systemic inflammation—considered a risk factor for cancer and cardiovascular diseases, among other conditions—is to measure the level of C-reactive protein in the blood. The liver naturally produces CRP in response to systemic inflammation. Research shows that about a third of US adults have systemic inflammation as measured by CRP,[1] but large portions of European and other populations are also affected—a consequence of normal aging and unhealthy behaviors, such as consumption of Western diets, obesity, and exposure to infection. Because the Mediterranean diet has been associated with a reduced risk of disease, many Europeans believe they are protected by their diet. Unfortunately, as I have shown in previous chapters, even the strictest form of the Mediterranean diet has a limited beneficial effect on aging and disease. And because most Europeans do not know what the

Mediterranean diet entails, and also because adherence to the strictest form is difficult, it is seldom adopted even in the Mediterranean region.

A recent worldwide analysis revealed that between 8 and 9 percent of the global population has been diagnosed with one of the major twenty-nine autoimmune diseases[2]—the most common being type 1 diabetes, multiple sclerosis, Crohn's disease, polymyalgia, psoriasis, lupus, and rheumatoid arthritis.

Alarmingly, the number of newly diagnosed cases of autoimmune diseases has been on the rise for the past thirty years. In the last decade, the incidence has jumped worldwide by a remarkable 19 percent a year.[3] In other words, autoimmune diseases appear to be doubling in number every five years. While some of this increase can be attributed to improved diagnosis and awareness of certain conditions, it's likely that environmental and dietary factors are also to blame.

Nutrition and Autoimmune Diseases

Obesity has been linked to multiple autoimmune diseases, including multiple sclerosis and rheumatoid arthritis. It may also be linked to Crohn's and other autoimmune diseases of the gut.[4] Because fat cells can be an important source of inflammatory molecules like TNF alpha and IL-6, the connection between obesity and autoimmune disorders could be related to abdominal fat. Fat accumulated in the abdomen and elsewhere in the body can generate molecules that stimulate immune responses, prompting immune cells to turn against other ordinary body cells.

High salt consumption is also believed to contribute to autoimmune diseases, possibly by promoting the activation of T cells—a central culprit in many autoimmune diseases. More studies are needed to confirm and understand the role of sodium in autoimmune disorders, but because salt is also involved in cardiovascular disease, moderation is generally recommended for those diagnosed with or at high risk for autoimmune diseases.

Diet can also affect the immune system by altering the bacteria population in the gut, which in turn regulates many different immune cells. It's well established that the Western diet can have inflammatory, negative effects on the types of microbiota occupying the human gut.[5] Research shows the bacterial population present in the gut of people eating an animal-based Western diet can be rapidly altered to a less inflammatory population simply by switching to a plant-based diet.[6]

At the Table with Your Ancestors

A less-understood potential factor explaining the rapid worldwide increase in autoimmune diseases may involve expanding choices in a modern, globalized food supply. My laboratory is only beginning to investigate this aspect of autoimmune diseases. We suspect, however, that certain aspects of today's globalized diet may trigger autoimmune responses. For example, in a study, cow's milk consumption in children was associated with elevated autoimmunity against the pancreatic cells that generate insulin, resulting in an increased risk for type 1 diabetes.[7] Eventually, it will be possible to connect a person's DNA (the genome) to the food he or she should avoid eating to prevent autoimmune disorders or intolerances. For now, my best advice is to "eat at the table of your ancestors."

This means finding out where your parents, grandparents, and great-grandparents came from and what foods were common in those places. My ancestors are all from Italy, and because of this my diet is rich in tomatoes, green beans, garbanzo beans, and olive oil. Tomatoes are known to activate an immune response in a small minority of people, and they arrived in Italy only four hundred years ago, but that's long enough that there is minimal risk that they will cause widespread autoimmunities or intolerances in today's Italians. In contrast, a grandchild of Japanese or southern Italians, both populations without milk in their traditional historical adult diet, is likely to develop lactose intolerance as an adult.

If my grandparents were from Okinawa, I would include sweet potatoes and seaweeds in my diet; if they were from Germany, cabbage and asparagus. It seems complicated, but it's not. It may require you to sit down with your parents or grandparents and ask questions, or ask an old person who used to live in the same area as your grandparents. Try to get the full list, since every component of their diet was probably selected to make up a full nourishment diet. Even though a little village like that of my parents in southern Italy did not conduct scientific studies to determine what diet was good or bad, everyone knew everyone else, and if someone developed vitamin B12 deficiency because they never ate fish or meat or eggs, everyone else in town would hear about it, and eventually learn how to avoid vitamin B12 deficiency. Similarly, if many babies who drank cow's milk developed problems, people would eventually notice and switch their babies to goat's milk. This type of food selection can happen more easily in villages and small towns, but it can also occur in cities if people live their whole lives in the same place. It would be much less likely to happen in the United States or in large cities like London or Tokyo, where communities are more transient and people know less about their neighbors' diseases and food habits.

We do not yet have solid evidence that "eating at the table of your ancestors" will prevent diseases and make you live longer. And I'm not proposing that you eat exactly what your grandparents ate, rather that you match what they ate with the Longevity Diet described in this book.

When you don't have the luxury of waiting until conclusive scientific and clinical studies are completed, it makes sense to adopt the best possible hypothesis using all the available information. In this case, the hypothesis is that a town of two thousand people and the surrounding towns—together with the doctors working in these towns—will be able to detect many of the advantages and disadvantages associated with particular foods by observing their effect over decades and by learning from their parents and grandparents. Much of the information will end up being correct. Some of it will be incorrect, but the risk of adopting this strategy is virtually zero—the food that was common and safe at the table of your ancestors is very unlikely to be harmful to you.

It's also important to know what your ancestors didn't eat. While the market may now be rich with so-called health foods and superfoods—ranging from kale to curcumin, quinoa to chia seeds—that can provide high levels of vitamins or protein, these varied ingredients and foods may be more harmful than helpful to people whose ancestors never consumed them. Quinoa, which originally comes from the Peruvian Andes, may be perfectly safe for people whose ancestors used it as a staple ingredient in their diet. It may also be fine for the great majority of people around the world. But it may lead to allergies, intolerances, and even autoimmune diseases in a small group of people—particularly those exposed to other factors contributing to autoimmune diseases. For example, quinoa was shown to increase the immune response in mice, which may be evidence of its potential to cause autoimmune diseases in humans,[8] and it was shown to cause severe allergic reactions in multiple patients in the United States and France.[9] Thus, if all your ancestors going back three hundred years lived in Germany, for example, it may be best to avoid "health foods" like quinoa and turmeric (curcumin), that historically were not key ingredients of the German diet.

Autoimmune Disease Treatment

The above-listed guidelines for the prevention of autoimmune diseases should also be adopted by patients undergoing disease treatment. In the following section, I focus on the use of FMD for the treatment of multiple sclerosis and rheumatoid arthritis—autoimmune diseases my group and others have investigated both in mouse studies and human clinical trials.

We have now tested the FMD with two additional major autoimmune diseases in mice. In both cases it worked surprisingly well, suggesting that FMD has the potential to reduce the severity of many autoimmune diseases. Please consider that these interventions are still under clinical or laboratory investigation and that, until larger clinical trials are completed, we cannot know whether they are effective in humans, nor can we exclude the possibility of severe side effects in a minority of patients.

Multiple Sclerosis

Multiple sclerosis (MS) is an autoimmune disorder in which immune cells (T cells) attack the insulating sheath around nerve fibers in the central nervous system. The clinical presentation

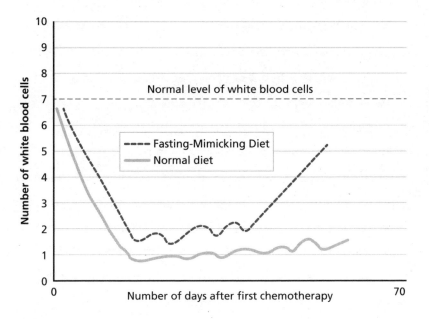

11.1. Fasting cycles regenerates immune cells after chemotherapy

includes debility of one or more limbs, partial or total loss of unilateral vision, and generalized pain. Patients generally suffer relapses of symptoms, which can be short but periodic. In some patients, the associated symptoms progress. Our research related to FMD and autoimmune diseases started after we discovered that fasting causes a major drop in the number of circulating white blood cells in mice, followed by a return to normal levels after they resume a normal diet (figure 11.1).[10]

In the same study, we showed that during fasting, long-term hematopoietic stem cells are turned on and expanded. This type of stem cell, found in the blood, is capable of generating the various cells of the immune system. Two research questions followed this finding:

1. Does the fasting preferentially kill dysfunctional cells, including autoimmune cells?
2. When animals or humans return to their normal diet after fasting, will the stem cells generate only healthy immune cells or will the new cells also become autoimmune?

After we published our findings, I started receiving emails from people who, having read media accounts of our study, had attempted fasting to fight their autoimmune disorders. Several reported to me that four or five days of FMD had reduced and in some cases even cured their autoimmune diseases.

The results of our first set of tests in mice were remarkable. To replace autoimmune cells with good ones, we hypothesized, we had to first kill off the bad ones. It worked. Cycles of the FMD not only reduced the severity of the multiple sclerosis in all mice; it

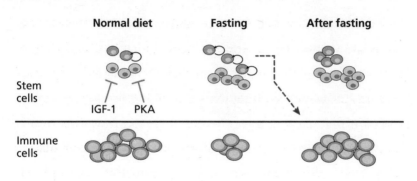

| Normal diet | Fasting | After fasting |

Stem cells

IGF-1   PKA

Immune cells

11.2. Rejuvenation from within

eliminated all symptoms in a portion of the mice that had already developed the disease. Each cycle of the FMD killed a portion of the autoimmune cells, and three cycles eliminated disease symptoms in 20 percent of the mice. FMD worked in another remarkable way: it promoted regeneration of the damaged myelin in the mouse spinal cord.

Thus, FMD cycles reversed the autoimmunity in a subset of mice by (1) killing off bad immune cells, (2) generating new and healthy ones, and (3) turning on progenitor cells (cells similar to stem cells), which can regenerate damaged nerves. This is an example of what I call "rejuvenation from within." FMD kills many cells, but it is particularly effective in killing off old and damaged immune cells that have lost the ability to distinguish between the cells of its own body and invading organisms such as bacteria and viruses. Fasting increases stem cells but reduces immune cells. After re-feeding, stem cells generate new and healthy immune cells (fig. 11.2).

In mice, FMD could do even more: it seemed to prompt the body to detect damage in the spinal cord—like it detects damage to the skin after a cut—and turn on stem and progenitor cells to repair the damage. Could the FMD actually cure multiple sclerosis in human patients?

In collaboration with other researchers, we performed a randomized clinical trial on patients with multiple sclerosis (relapsing-remitting) to determine just this.[11] Twenty MS patients were asked to undergo a single seven-day cycle of an FMD, followed by a Mediterranean diet for six months. The choice of the Mediterranean diet instead of the Longevity Diet was made by our clinical collaborators at Charité–University Medicine Berlin. In our future MS studies, we anticipate combining the periodic FMD with the everyday Longevity Diet. A control group of twenty MS patients continued their normal diet.

The FMD began with a pre-fasting day of 800 calories from fruit, rice, and/or potatoes. This was followed by seven fasting days, during which patients consumed 200 to 350 calories a day from vegetable broths or vegetable juice, supplemented with linseed oil (omega-3) three times daily. Patients were advised to drink 2 to 3 liters of unsweetened fluids each day (water and herbal teas). After the seven-day FMD period, solid foods were reintroduced slowly for three days. Patients followed a plant-based Mediterranean diet for the next six months (see chapter 4). An additional twenty MS patients were placed on a "ketogenic diet" (very high levels of fat, normal protein, and low carbohydrates) for six months; a ketogenic diet had previously shown improved outcomes for MS patients.

After the study ended, patients who had received a single cycle of FMD reported significant improvements in quality of life, physical health, and mental health. Side effects unrelated to MS were similar in both groups and were reported by approximately 20 percent of patients on the regular diet and those receiving the FMD. The most common side effects were respiratory tract infections and urinary tract infections, but there was no indication of liver or other damage. Ninety percent of the patients in the FMD group were able to complete the trial period. During the six-month study period, four relapses were observed in the control group, and three relapses were observed in the FMD group.

Overall, this study indicates that FMD is safe and potentially effective in MS patients, although additional and larger studies are necessary to confirm these results. Notably, whereas mice received multiple cycles of FMD, human subjects received only one seven-day cycle, which raises the possibility that efficacy would increase once multiple cycles are tested in human MS patients, followed by the Longevity Diet. We are now preparing to perform several larger clinical trials with hundreds of MS patients exposed to multiple cycles of FMD.

Crohn's Disease and Colitis

After we published our work on fasting and immunity, journalist and autoimmune disease sufferer Jenni Russell of the *Times* of London wrote several articles about it. I include one of these articles below. At the time, it was too early to tell journalists about our work on multiple sclerosis and other autoimmune disorders, but we were already convinced the results were promising.

Fasting Transformed Me
After Medicine Failed

BY JENNI RUSSELL

Times of London | *April 22, 2015*

In the last ten months, my life has been transformed. I didn't write a book, move house, have children, find a faith, or change my job. Instead, I have gone from being an exhausted person with a lifelong and incurable illness, kept alive by four drugs, to a currently healthy and energetic one. This remarkable difference has been brought about by a therapy that's simple, free and overlooked by the NHS: fasting.

I tried fasting because I was desperate. It's two decades since I developed a serious autoimmune condition which has often left me sleeping 12 hours a day and sometimes kept me in bed for months at a time. It was made worse by chemotherapy for cancer five years ago. I was told after that I could never live without immune-suppressing drugs; when I tried to, I was rushed to hospital as an emergency admission and spent several days on drips.

That was when I came across research from the University of Southern California. Valter Longo, a leading biogerontologist who had been studying the effects of fasting on mice for 20 years, had discovered that if mice were starved for three days, their immune systems started to regenerate. Starvation forced the bone marrow to create stem cells, replacing the faulty immune response with a normal one. Intermittent fasts over six months created steady improvement. This therapy might, said Longo, prove remarkably effective for anyone with an autoimmune condition or whose immune system was deteriorating with age. He cautioned that nothing was proven until human trials had been done.

I had nothing to lose by trying it, except my temper and

a little weight. I started the first fast on a boat journey on a stormy sea. It was made a lot easier by the fact that I'd lost my appetite anyway, and that I wasn't required to do anything except lie in a bunk and read. Still, it was very boring to have nothing to look forward to but hot water, cold water, fizzy water; black tea, green tea, mint tea. I got fiercely hungry, and sometimes dizzy, but the sensation would pass. I lasted two and a half days and thought nothing could come of it. On the fourth day, I woke feeling better than I had for years.

Since then I have fasted three more times, most recently for four days. It's no fun. I couldn't do it while working, or cooking for anyone else. You need to be free to crash out whenever your indignant body complains. You also need distractions to look forward to when you remember, gloomily, that there isn't a meal ahead; books, films, the company of partners and friends.

I only do it because the results have been so dramatic. I am off every drug, and for the first time since getting ill I don't have to ration my energy and time. I can't know if it will last, but I have become a quiet evangelist. Fasting, as one doctor said recently, may be the panacea that western medicine forgot.

In the last few years diabetes researchers have found that the disease can be cured by a daily 600-calorie diet for eight weeks. Longo's own earlier research indicates that fasting is as effective as chemotherapy in treating cancer. Combining the two, fasting just before and after treatment, increases the efficacy of chemo by up to 40 per cent while minimizing side-effects. Cancer cells cope badly with being simultaneously poisoned and starved. But normal cells gain protection, because fasting closes the pathways that let toxins in. Since a fifth of all cancer-related deaths are due to the effects of chemo, this may be a major breakthrough.

We have now carried out mouse studies on Crohn's disease. The results are not yet published, but I can confirm they are very promising. Patients suffering from Crohn's, colitis, or another gastrointestinal inflammatory disease should talk to their doctors about using an FMD in support of standard-of-care therapy. If the neurologist agrees, follow the FMD protocol in our multiple sclerosis article[12] once every two months until either the symptoms improve or it becomes clear that the diet does not help. It is best if this is done as part of a clinical trial.

Rheumatoid Arthritis

Rheumatoid arthritis is a chronic autoimmune inflammatory disease resulting in the destruction of multiple joints. It affects about 1 percent of the overall population and 2 percent of people over the age of sixty. Fasting or very low-calorie diets lasting one to three weeks have been shown to be effective in the treatment of rheumatoid arthritis, or RA. Inflammation and pain typical of RA can improve within a few days of commencing the fast,[13] but they return after patients resume their normal diet. If the fasting period is followed by a vegetarian diet, some of the therapeutic effects remain.[14] This combination therapy has produced beneficial results lasting years.[15] The efficacy of this approach has been confirmed by four different studies, including two randomized clinical trials.[16] For many patients able to endure long-term fasting and willing to permanently modify their diet, fasting cycles have the potential to not only augment but also replace existing medical treatments.[17]

What has yet to be tried is multiple/periodic cycles of the periodic FMD every one to three months in the treatment of RA instead of a single cycle followed by major changes in the diet. Our research on multiple sclerosis, Crohn's, and several other autoimmune diseases—combined with our clinical results suggesting that FMD reduces systemic inflammation in the great majority of patients with high inflammation (CRP) at the beginning of the trial—suggests that the ideal way to treat RA will be with cycles of the five-day FMD (see chapter 6) every one to three months. Between cycles, I recommend the Longevity Diet described in chapter 4. We have evidence that monthly cycles of FMD could benefit RA patients even in the absence of switching to a Mediterranean or Longevity Diet. While this is not my recommendation, for those who cannot permanently change their diet, the monthly five days of FMD may be a good option. Notably, FMD would have the advantage of providing relatively high calories, which would allow patients to do this under medical supervision but without checking into a clinic. Considering that in our pilot multiple sclerosis trial a weeklong FMD was safe and potentially effective in improving patients' quality of life, and considering past studies on RA, a periodic seven-day FMD may be more effective than a shorter one. After future studies, we will know more about the efficacy of FMD against various autoimmune disorders. We will also know more about the length and frequency of the diet best suited to treating these diseases.

Summary: Prevention and Treatment of Autoimmune Diseases

Prevention

1. Follow the Longevity Diet, making sure you do so in such a way that you maintain a healthy weight and low abdominal circumference.
2. Avoid a high-salt diet.
3. Eat foods your ancestors ate frequently, and avoid foods that were not part of their diet.

Treatment

1. Adopt all changes in the "Prevention" section above.
2. With your doctor's approval and close supervision, and preferably as part of a clinical trial, alternate the Longevity Diet with a monthly five-day FMD, or the seven-day FMD described above every *two* months.

Chapter 12

How to Stay Young

I'VE POSTPONED WRITING THIS BOOK for years out of concern that my recommendations, while optimizing healthy longevity, would cause side effects. Before I could put this down on paper, I needed to determine how nutrients are linked to genes and molecules in cells, mice, and people, and to understand whether and how the body can fix and rejuvenate itself. I had to test my theory on myself and in randomized clinical trials. I also followed thousands of patients with cancer, diabetes, multiple sclerosis, and other diseases and conditions as part of clinical trials or often directly by working with them or with their physicians. I performed parallel studies of human populations with specific genetic mutations, such as the Laron's community in Ecuador, and consumed specific diets, such as the centenarians in Calabria and Okinawa. Finally, I performed epidemiological studies of large US populations to understand the association between the consumption of certain foods and disease.

I am grateful to the extraordinary students and research scientists in my laboratories in Los Angeles and Milan who have given their all for years, allowing me to test and prove my hypotheses. I am also grateful to my collaborators from all parts of the globe and across many fields of study. In the thirty years that I have worked on aging, the motivation driving me forward was the desire to discover the genes and molecular mechanisms that regulate aging and a healthy lifespan with the final goal to help people who have run out of therapeutic options. Not long ago I visited a famous journalist in the end stages of cancer. His oncologists had shrugged and sent him home.

"There's nothing more we can do," they told him.

Although I understand why his doctors were reluctant to try out my ideas—he had lost so much weight by the time I met him—I actually believe there is almost always something that can be done. Unfortunately, the system is not always set up to allow this. Sadly, I wasn't able to intervene in his case, and he has since passed away. I don't know what would have happened to the Air France pilot, the judge in Los Angeles, or the *Times* journalist if they had not tried fasting-based diets, but I suspect they would not have done as well as they did. At the same time, there is an official and appropriate process of identifying medical interventions (large randomized trials, FDA approval, etc.), that is as important as trying new and creative interventions and which cannot be ignored. Thus, when there are no viable options, it is important to adopt a therapeutic compromise that is respectful of the official methods but which carefully considers integrative therapies based on sufficient scientific and safety data.

I am confident, thanks to evidence from the Five Pillars, that our FMD and other nutritional and integrative approaches will continue to help people remain healthy and/or become healthier by acting on the ability of the body to regenerate and rejuvenate itself. I also hope our longevity studies, and others coming out of my colleagues' labs, will bring swift implementation by medical doctors and dietitians who are in a position to act on new, proven, low-cost integrative treatments.

My favorite novel is Luigi Pirandello's *One, None and One Hundred Thousand*. The book's premise is marvelously simple: If no one knows you, in some way, you don't exist; but if one hundred thousand people know you, there are one hundred thousand versions of you living in their heads. I see our work in the same way. If we make a discovery that helps no one, then in a way we haven't discovered anything at all. But if our discovery helps a hundred thousand people live longer and healthier, then our discoveries live in the people who are alive or healthier because of them.

So I hope that this book will sell as well in the rest of the world as it has sold in Italy, not only because I hope that it will help many people reach old age in good health, but also because 100 percent of my royalties from the sale will be donated to support our continued multidisciplinary studies.

Below, I briefly summarize the most important findings and conclusions of our research.

1. **Eat a mostly vegan diet with some fish:** Strive for a 100 percent plant- and fish-based diet, but limit fish consumption to two or three meals a week and avoid fish with high mercury content. After age sixty-five to seventy, if you start losing muscle mass, strength, and weight, add more fish and fruit and introduce animal-based foods like eggs, cheese, and yogurt made from sheep's or goat's milk.

2. **Consume low but sufficient proteins:** Consume approximately 0.31 to 0.36 grams of protein per pound of body weight per day. If you weigh 100 pounds, that is about 31 to 36 grams of protein per day, of which 30 grams should be consumed in a single meal to maximize muscle synthesis. If you weigh 200 pounds and have 35 percent body fat, 60 grams of protein per day are instead sufficient, considering that it is the lean body mass that utilizes most of the proteins. Protein intake should be raised slightly after age sixty-five to seventy in individuals who are losing weight and muscle.

3. **Minimize bad fats and sugars, and maximize good fats and complex carbs:** The diet should be rich in "good" unsaturated fats, including those from salmon, almonds, and walnuts, but very poor in "bad" saturated, hydrogenated, and trans fats. Likewise, the diet should be rich in complex carbohydrates, such as those provided by whole bread and vegetables, but poor in sugars and limited in pasta, rice, white bread, fruit juices, and fruits containing carbohydrates that are eas-

ily converted into simple sugars. Finally, the diet should be low in animal proteins but relatively high in vegetable proteins, in order to minimize the former's negative effects on diseases and maximize the latter's nourishing effects.

4. **Be nourished:** The body needs protein, essential fatty acids (omega-3 and omega-6), minerals, vitamins, and sufficient sugar to fight the many wars going on inside and outside cells. To be sure you get enough nutrients, every three days take a multivitamin and a mineral pill, plus an omega-3 fish oil soft gel purchased from a reputable manufacturer.

5. **Eat at the table of your ancestors:** Consume a variety of foods to take in all the required nutrients, but choose the ones that were common on the table of your parents, grandparents, and great-grandparents, so long as they are included in the Longevity Diet.

6. **Eat twice a day plus a snack:** Unless your waist circumference and body weight are in the normal or low range, it is best to eat breakfast plus one other meal a day and one low-calorie, low-sugar, nourishing snack. If your weight or muscle mass is too low, then eat three meals a day plus a snack.

7. **Time-restricted eating:** Restrict your eating to eleven to twelve hours or less per day. For example, if you eat breakfast after 8 a.m., finish dinner before 8 p.m. Shorter periods of feeding (ten hours or less) have been shown to be even more effective in promoting health, but they are much more diffi-

cult to comply with and may increase the risk of side effects, such as the formation of gallstones.

8. **Periodic prolonged fasting-mimicking diets:** People who are under seventy years of age, not frail or malnourished, and free of certain diseases should undergo five-day periods during which they consume a relatively high-calorie fasting-mimicking diet (see chapter 6). An FMD may also be appropriate for older people, but only if needed and if a medical doctor recommends it.

9. Follow steps 1 through 8 in such a way that you reach and maintain a waist circumference of less than 35.5 inches for men and less than 29.5 inches for women. This is higher than the ideal 33 inches and 27 inches cited earlier, but it is more realistic and should still be very effective in reducing disease risk while avoiding malnourishment.

Exercise for Longevity

Walk fast one hour per day. Take the stairs instead of escalators and elevators, even if you have to go up many flights. On the weekend, try to walk, even to faraway places, but avoid polluted areas. Do moderate exercise for 2.5 hours a week, some of it in the vigorous range. Do weight training or weight-free exercises to strengthen muscles (combined with 30 grams of protein intake following the weight training).

A Long-Lived Mind

I have written very little in this book about the mind. I am not an expert in this area, and I find that studies investigating how the mind can help us live longer and healthier are few and inconclusive. Although there are many studies on social aspects of longevity, it would be difficult to find a set of consistent basic, clinical, epidemiological, and centenarian studies supporting a major role for a particular social behavior in healthy longevity. In the absence of strong scientific data, I surmise that staying close to family members and friends, belonging to religious or spiritual organizations, and volunteering to help others are all important to a long and healthy life. However, I have also seen many lonely people live long and healthy lives, probably because they focus on simple pleasures and obtain strength from their own instincts and ability to find happiness in little things—eating certain foods, walking in the park, talking to the cashier at the local grocery store. My father, who is ninety-one, recently had part of his stomach removed because of a suspected tumor. He is separated from my mother and lives alone. His recovery was difficult, and he was losing weight for several weeks. So he started eating chocolate and other treats he had enjoyed in his youth but had not indulged in for many years. He resumed a daily exercise regimen. He not only regained the weight he had lost, but he also sounded happier when we spoke and looked forward to each day. Making it to 110 in good health, in my father's case, is less about social connections and great friendships and more about simple things, like that long-forbidden chocolate bar. In the case of Salvatore Caruso, who watched my father grow up, it was about competition. He wanted to be the oldest man in the world. When I informed him that someone in Sicily was older, he said: "I have to beat him." And he eventually did.

Salvatore, someday I hope to beat you. I'll see you on the other side, old friend. I hope it's a very long time from now.

Appendix A:
Longevity Diet
Two-Week Meal Plan*

THE FOLLOWING TWO-WEEK MEAL PLAN IS based on the Longevity Diet described in chapter 4. These recipes reflect the types of ingredients and combinations most beneficial to your health. Feel free to substitute equivalent ingredients while maintaining a similar nutrient composition. For example, when a recipe calls for pasta, you may replace it with whole-wheat pasta, barley, farro, semolina, polenta, gnocchi, or wild rice, keeping the portion within the suggested 40-gram serving. This dietary plan was developed to maximize required levels of vitamins and minerals without interfering with other longevity-promoting food components. Incorporate as many as possible of the ingredients listed in the vitamins, minerals, and other micronutrient tables (see appendix B). These are excellent sources of vitamins and minerals

---

* This section was written in collaboration with nutritionist Noemi Renzetti and dietitians Mahshid Shelechi and Susan Kim.

commonly deficient in the Western diet: vitamin B12, vitamin D, folate, vitamin A, vitamin C, vitamin E, calcium, iron, magnesium, and omega-3 (from fish oil or other sources). To prevent deficiencies, I encourage you to take a complete multivitamin and mineral pill and one omega-3 oil soft gel every three days. This diet is ideal for people of normal weight, ages twenty to sixty-five years. After age sixty-five, calorie and protein intake should be adjusted up to prevent unwanted weight and muscle loss.

The following diet consists of three meals (breakfast, lunch, and dinner) and one snack. It provides approximately 1,700 to 1,800 calories per day. This is the average calorie requirement for a sedentary woman of normal height (5 feet, 4 inches), weight (125 pounds), and body mass index (21.5) between the ages of thirty-one and fifty, or a moderately active woman over age fifty-one. Men of normal height (5 feet, 8 inches), weight (152 pounds), and BMI (22.5) should increase every ingredient in these recipes by approximately 20 percent. The portion sizes should be adjusted based on the need to maintain or reach a normal body weight (BMI and abdominal circumference; see chapter 4). Those who tend to lose weight and drop below the normal range may increase the portions of various dishes, while those who tend to gain weight may decrease them or combine lunch and dinner while reducing portion sizes. The diet provides approximately 55 to 60 percent of calories from carbohydrates, with most coming in the ideal complex-carbohydrate form contained in vegetables and grains, but also in pasta and bread. There are virtually no components with sugar added, although sugar is present in fruit and other foods. The diet provides approximately 30 to 35 percent of calories from fats, the great majority of which are in the form of "healthy" unsaturated fats, and 10 to 11 percent of calories from proteins, with the great majority coming from plants and fish.

The lunches and dinners are grouped into one low-calorie, low-protein meal and one high-calorie, high-protein meal providing all the necessary nutrients. The high-calorie, high-protein meal contains at least 30 grams of protein to optimize muscle growth (see chapter 5). Although low-protein meals are listed as lunches, they can be switched with dinners. However, I recommend using the low-protein meals either for all the lunches or for all the dinners. All meals should be consumed within a daily twelve-hour window, and the last meal should be consumed at least three to four hours before bedtime.

Important Notice

Remember that the calories you consume need to be adjusted according to your basal metabolic rate (BMR) and daily physical activity level (PAL). To calculate your ideal daily protein intake, multiply your body weight in kilograms by 0.8 (USDA, 2016; ISTAT, 2015; WHO, 2015). Achieving balance between calories consumed and calories burned through daily physical activity is essential to maintaining an ideal body weight and maximum health. Consuming just 150 calories a day beyond what your body needs can lead to ten pounds of extra body weight gained in twelve months. Note that the energy content and nutritional values of any food component listed in the following diet may differ depending on the types and brands you choose.

References (Diet)

"Balance Food and Activity." Bethesda, MD: National Institutes of Health, 2016. Available from http://www.nhlbi.nih.gov/health/educational/wecan/healthy-weight-basics/balance.htm.

Country statistics: Italy. Geneva: World Health Organization, 2016. Available from http://www.who.int/countries/ita/en.

Food and Nutrition Information Center. "Interactive DRI [Dietary Reference Intakes] for Professionals." Washington, DC: United States Department of Agriculture, 2016. Available from http://fnic.nal.usda.gov/fnic/interactiveDRI/index.php.

Guideline: Sugars Intake for Adults and Children. Geneva: World Health Organization, 2015. Available from http://apps.who.int/iris/bitstream/10665/149782/1/9789241549028_eng.pdf?ua=1.

Italia in cifre (Italy in figures). Rome: Istituto Nazionale di Statistica, 2015: Available from http://www.istat.it/it/files/2015/08/ItaliaInCifre2015It.pdf.

WEEK 1*

DAY 1

Breakfast

Coffee, espresso or American; barley (no caffeine) is an acceptable alternative

---

* Portions are calculated for a woman of average weight, of average height, and with a BMI of 21.5. Men of normal weight and height may increase portions by 20 percent. Portions should be based on your ability to reach and maintain a normal weight and BMI, and on your desire to either lose or gain weight. I recommend daily weight and abdominal-circumference measurements (see chapter 4) until the ideal weight is reached and stabilized.

Almond, hazelnut, or coconut milk, unsweetened and
supplemented with calcium and vitamins B12, B2, and D
(1 glass, 240 mL)

Whole-wheat focaccia and extra virgin olive oil (60 g)

Blueberry jam, no sugar added (20 g, 1 tbsp)

Lunch

Spinach with pine nuts and raisins

INGREDIENTS:

Spinach (150 g)

Pine nuts (9 g, 1 tbsp)

Raisins (9 g, 1 tbsp)

Olive oil (12 mL, 1 tbsp)

Salt to taste*

Spelt crackers (40 g)

Boil the spinach in water. Drain the water and mix the
cooked spinach with the pine nuts and raisins. Cook for a
few minutes on a pan, adding water to avoid drying. Turn
off the heat, add oil, stir and let the mixture rest, covered,
for 2 to 3 minutes. Crackers to be consumed on the side.

Snack

Coconut milk, unsweetened (1 glass, 240 mL)

Nut and whole-grain dark chocolate bar; choose a brand
containing 150 calories, low in sugar (less than 8 g), made
with 70% minimum dark chocolate and no milk

---

* US Dietary Guidelines recommend limiting sodium to less than 2.3 grams
a day.

Dinner

Pasta with broccoli and black beans

Black beans, boiled (150 g wet,* drained)

Broccoli, boiled (200 g)

Pasta, whole grain (40 g)

Olive oil (25 mL, 2 tbsp)

Garlic (1 clove), sliced thinly

Hot pepper

Salt and pepper to taste

Parmesan cheese (5 g, 1 tbsp)

Bring a large pot of water to boil. Add salt, the black beans, broccoli, and pasta. Cook until the pasta is ready. Drain and toss with the olive oil, garlic, hot pepper, and Parmesan cheese.

Suggested dessert:[†] walnuts (25 g) and unsweetened dried cranberries (20 g) or other unsweetened dried fruit

Take a complete multivitamin and mineral pill and one omega-3 oil soft gel.

---

* Throughout these recipes, when possible use fresh and seasonal vegetables, and dried legumes (beans, lentils, peas) that have been soaked overnight.

† Sugar is naturally present in fruits and dried fruits. In the following daily meal plans, limit added sugar (to sweeten coffee or tea) and sugar naturally present in fruit juices, honey, and syrups to less than 8 to 10 grams a day (2 teaspoons).

DAY 2

Breakfast

Tea with fresh-squeezed lemon (use 2 teabags: 1 green tea and
1 black tea)

Cereal (60 g) with almond milk (240 mL)

Lunch

Wild rice and green beans with garlic and fresh tomato

Wild rice (40 g)

Green beans (150 g)

Fresh tomato (150 g)

Garlic (2 cloves)

Salt (add based on taste, trying to keep as low as possible)

Olive oil (12 mL, 1 tbsp)

Lemon

Fresh basil

Pepper

Cook the wild rice. In a separate pot, cover the green beans
with water and add the tomato, garlic, and salt. When the
beans are tender, add the oil and basil and let them rest for
2 to 3 minutes before serving over the rice.

Side dish: leafy green vegetables (e.g., chicory or kale),
boiled and seasoned with olive oil and lemon (200 g)

Snack

Hazelnut milk, unsweetened (1 glass, 240 mL)

Nut and whole-grain dark chocolate bar; choose a brand containing 150 calories, low in sugar (less than 8 g), made with 70% minimum dark chocolate and no milk

Dinner

Salmon fillet (wild caught) with asparagus

Salmon fillet (150 g)

Asparagus (300 g)

Olive oil (12 mL, 1 tbsp)

Lemon juice to taste

Salt and pepper to taste

Whole-wheat bread (60 g) (to be consumed on the side)

Steam or bake the salmon fillet and asparagus. Serve drizzled with the olive oil and seasoned with lemon and salt and pepper.

Side dish: mixed green salad with tomatoes, carrots, fennel, and green peppers seasoned with balsamic vinegar (200 g)

Suggested dessert: hazelnuts (25 g) and dried cranberries (30 g)

DAY 3

Breakfast

> Coffee or tea
>
> Whole-wheat bread, toasted (60 g)
>
> Mixed berry jam, no sugar added (40 g, 2 tsp)

Lunch

> Spelt and zucchini with garlic, olives, and parsley

> > Spelt (40 g)
> >
> > Zucchini (300 g)
> >
> > Garlic (1 clove)
> >
> > Cut cherry tomatoes (100 g)
> >
> > Olives (25 g)
> >
> > Parsley
> >
> > Olive oil (12 mL, 1 tbsp)
> >
> > Salt

> Boil the spelt in salted water. Drain and set it aside. In a separate pan, boil the zucchini with the garlic, cherry tomatoes, and olives. When the zucchini is tender, drain the water, stir in the parsley, the cooked rice , and the olive oil. Let it rest for 2 to 3 minutes before serving.

> *Side dish:* green leafy vegetables (e.g., Swiss chard), boiled and seasoned with oil and lemon (200 g)

Snack

Garbanzo bean bread (*farinata di ceci*) with raw vegetables
(e.g., carrots and/or celery); or fresh mixed-berry
smoothie (150 g) with hazelnut milk (125 mL)

Garbanzo bean flour (240 g)

Water (240 mL)

Olive oil (2 tbsp, optional)

Pinch of salt and pepper

To make this gluten-free bread—a typical recipe from
Liguria, Italy—place the garbanzo bean flour in a bowl
and add the water and oil. Whisk until smooth. Pour the
batter in a metal pie pan and bake in a preheated 350°F
oven until edges begin to brown (about 15 minutes). Alter-
natively, cook the farinata in a pan over medium heat.
Sprinkle with salt and pepper.

Dinner

Garbanzo bean minestrone with pasta

Mixed minestrone vegetables (250 g)

Garbanzo beans (150 g wet weight)

Pasta (40 g)

Olive oil (25 mL, 2 tbsp)

Salt and pepper (keep salt as low as possible)

Parmesan cheese (5 g, 1 tbsp)

Bring a large pot of water to a boil. Add salt, the mixed
vegetables, and soaked garbanzo beans. When the vegetables are tender, add the pasta. When pasta is cooked, drain

and add the olive oil. Serve the soup sprinkled with Parmesan cheese.

Side dish: mixed green salad with tomatoes, carrots, fennel, and green peppers, seasoned with olive oil and lemon

Suggested dessert: cherries (100 g) or dried cherries (20 g) and almonds (25 g)

WEEK 1

DAY 4

Breakfast

Coffee or tea (with ½ squeezed lemon)

Cinnamon raisin bagel or 2 pieces of toast (80 g)

Apricot jam, no sugar added (20 g, 1 tbsp)

Lunch

Barley salad with olives and nuts

Barley (40 g)

Tomatoes (150 g)

Mushrooms, raw (75 g)

Peppers, raw (150 g)

Corn (20 g)

Pickled vegetables: artichokes, cucumber, and spring onions (150 g)

Pecans (9 g)

Olives (12 g, 1 tbsp)

Olive oil (12 mL, 1 tbsp)

Salt and pepper to taste

Other herbs (optional)

Boil the barley in salted water following the package in-structions. Cut the tomatoes, mushrooms, peppers, and corn into a salad bowl. Add the pickled vegetables, pecans, and olives. Season in water with salt and pepper, and/or other herbs. When the barley is ready, let it cool briefly before adding it to the prepared mix. Add the olive oil. Serve it warm or store it in the refrigerator to enjoy as a fresh summer dish.

Snack

Coconut milk, unsweetened (1 glass, 240 mL)

Nut and whole-grain dark chocolate bar; choose a brand containing 150 calories, low in sugar (less than 8 g), made with 70% minimum dark chocolate and no milk

Dinner

Pasta and lentil soup (*pasta e lenticchie*)

Lentils (150 g drained)

Potato (1 medium)

Carrot (1 medium)

Tomato (1 medium)

Garlic (2 cloves, cut in half)

Rosemary (as desired)

Pasta (40 g)

Olive oil (25 mL, 2 tbsp)

Boil the soaked lentils in a large pot of salted water with the potato, carrot, tomato, garlic, and rosemary. When the lentils are tender, add the pasta. When pasta is cooked, stir, and let the water evaporate until the soup reaches the desired consistency. Turn fire off, and add olive oil.

Suggested dessert: pineapple (100 g) or dried blueberries (20 g) and walnuts (25 g)

Take a complete multivitamin and mineral pill and one omega-3 oil soft gel.

WEEK 1

DAY 5

Breakfast

Coffee, espresso or American
Oats, steel cut (90 g)

> Oats, steel cut (90 g)
> Almond milk (1 glass, 240 mL)
> Honey (10 g, 2 tsp)
> Fresh fruit (e.g., 1 medium banana and 1 kiwi)

Cook the oats in water for 30 minutes. Let them cool. Add honey and fresh fruit.

Lunch

Escarole, olives, tomatoes, and basil

> Escarole (150 g)
> Pine nuts (9 g, 1 tbsp)
> Olive oil (12 mL, 1 tbsp)
> Sun-dried tomatoes (150 g)

Basil (5 leaves)

Brown bread, toasted (40 g) (on the side)

Boil the escarole. Drain and allow it to cool slightly. Add the olive oil, sun-dried tomatoes, olives, and basil.

Side dish: fresh carrots (150 g), raw (seasoned with oil, salt, and lemon) or boiled in water (seasoned with oil, salt, and pepper)

Snack

Hazelnut milk, unsweetened (1 glass, 240 mL)

Nut and whole-grain dark chocolate bar; choose a brand containing 150 calories, low in sugar (less than 8 g), made with 70% minimum dark chocolate and no milk

Dinner

Octopus with potato (*polpo e patate schiacciate*)

Octopus, fresh or frozen (60 g)

Potato (1 medium)

Cherry tomatoes (150 g)

Olives (20 g)

Olive oil (25 mL, 2 tbsp)

Parsley

Lemon

Salt

Brown bread, toasted (40 g)

Boil the octopus and potato in separate saucepans. Drain both. Cut the octopus and mash the boiled potato in a bowl. Add the cherry tomatoes, olives, and oil. Season with lemon, parsley, and salt.

Side dish: mixed green salad with cucumber, tomatoes, and carrots, seasoned with balsamic vinegar (200 g)

Suggested dessert: cranberries (50 g) or dried cranberries (20 g) and almonds (25 g)

WEEK 1

DAY 6

Breakfast

Coffee or tea (with ½ squeezed lemon)

Whole-wheat dried focaccia with olive oil (60 g)

Fresh fruit (1 apple and strawberries)

Lunch

Grilled eggplant with feta cheese and tomatoes

Eggplant (250 g)

Olive oil (12 mL, 1 tbsp)

Cherry tomatoes (150 g)

Feta cheese (20 g)

Basil

Salt and pepper

Rye crackers (40 g)

Slice and grill the eggplant. When the slices are tender, place them in a heated pan with the olive oil, cherry tomatoes, and feta cheese. Season with basil and salt and pepper.

Cover and let it rest for 2 to 3 minutes. Serve with the rye crackers.

Snack

Almond milk, unsweetened (1 glass, 240 mL)

Nut and whole-grain dark chocolate bar; choose a brand containing 150 calories, low in sugar (less than 8 g), made with 70% minimum dark chocolate and no milk

Dinner

Pasta e vaianeia (Molochio recipe, see chapter 4)

Navy beans (150 g, wet, drained)

Green beans (150 g)

Carrots (2 medium), sliced

Potato (1 medium, cubed)

Zucchini (150 g), sliced

Tomato (1 large)

Garlic (2 cloves, cut in half)

Basil (5 leaves)

Pasta (40 g)

Olive oil (25 mL, 2 tbsp)

Salt to taste

Parmesan cheese (5 g, 1 tbsp)

Bring water to boil in a large pan. Add salt and the soaked navy beans. When the beans are tender, add the cut green beans and carrots. Boil the mixture for 30 minutes, then add the potato and boil for another 15 minutes. Add the zucchini and boil for 5 minutes. Add the whole tomato, boil it until tender, then smash it and remove its skin from the pot. Add the garlic, basil, and pasta. When pasta is cooked, add the olive oil, salt, and pepper. Stir until evenly mixed and heated through.

Side dish: mixed green salad with tomatoes, carrots, corn, and cucumber, seasoned with oil and lemon

Suggested dessert: hazelnuts (25 g) and dried blueberries (20 g)

WEEK 1

DAY 7
Breakfast
Coffee, espresso or American

Almond milk (1 glass, 240 mL)

Fruit and nut cereal (60 g)

Fresh fruit (1 medium)

Lunch
Brussels sprouts with garlic, pine nuts, and Parmesan cheese

Brussels sprouts (250 g)

Garlic (2 cloves, sliced)

Pine nuts (9 g, 1 tsp)

Hot pepper (optional)

Olive oil (12 mL, 1 tbsp)

Parmesan cheese (5 g, 1 tbsp)

Salt and pepper

Dark whole-grain bread (40 g) (on the side)

Boil the brussels sprouts in salted water. Drain, reserving a little of the cooking water. Transfer the sprouts and reserved water to a heated pan. Add the garlic, pine nuts, and hot pepper, stirring for 2 to 3 minutes. Let the mixture rest. Add the olive oil. Sprinkle with Parmesan cheese and add salt and pepper to taste.

Side dish: mixed green salad with red peppers, tomatoes, carrots, and mushrooms (200 g total), seasoned with vinegar

Snack

Goat's milk yogurt (125 g)

Nut and whole-grain dark chocolate bar; choose a brand containing 150 calories, low in sugar (less than 8 g), made with 70% minimum dark chocolate and no milk

Dinner

Spaghetti with clams and mussels

Clams and mussels (60 g total)
Garlic (2 cloves)
Tomato, chopped
Parsley (based on taste)
White cooking wine (40 mL)
Spaghetti (40 g)
Olive oil (25 mL, 2 tbsp)
Salt and pepper

Cook the clams and mussels in a pan with water and the garlic, tomato, parsley, and cooking wine. In a separate pot, boil the spaghetti in salted water. Drain the pasta and place it in the pan with the cooked clams and mussels. While the pan is still hot, stir in the olive oil. Add salt and pepper to taste. Serve with fresh parsley.

Side dish: leafy green vegetables, boiled and seasoned with oil, salt, and pepper

Suggested dessert: dates (20 g) and walnuts (25 g)

Take a complete multivitamin and mineral pill and one omega-3 oil soft gel.

WEEK 2

DAY 1

Breakfast

Coffee or tea (with ½ squeezed lemon)
Oats with almond milk, chocolate, nuts, and berries

Oats, steel cut (80 g)
Almond milk (1 glass, 240 mL)
Fresh mixed berries (150 g)

Cook the oats in water for 30 minutes. Remove them from heat, mix in the dark chocolate, nuts, and berries.

Lunch

Greek salad with feta, olives, onion, and peppers

Mixed lettuce (150 g)
Feta cheese (20 g)

Peppers, green and red (200 g)

Cherry tomatoes (150 g)

Onion (optional)

Olives (20 g)

Olive oil (12 mL, 1 tbsp)

Salt to taste

Brown bread (40 g) (on the side)

Snack

Hazelnut milk, unsweetened (1 glass, 240 mL)

Nut and whole-grain dark chocolate bar; choose a brand
containing 150 calories, low in sugar (less than 8 g), made
with 70% minimum dark chocolate and no milk

Dinner

Garbanzo bean salad and vegetables with garbanzo bean
bread

Garbanzo beans (150 g), cooked or canned (drained)

Onion (1 medium), chopped

Olive oil (25 mL, 2 tbsp)

Salt and pepper to taste

Spinach, boiled (200 g)

Lemon juice

Garbanzo bean bread (60 g) (recipe, page 228)

Season the garbanzo beans with the onion, olive oil, and
salt and pepper. Boil the spinach separately in salted water.
Add the spinach to the seasoned garbanzo beans, adding

more oil and lemon juice as needed. Serve with garbanzo bean bread.

Suggested dessert: pecan nuts (25 g) and dates (20 g)

WEEK 2

DAY 2

Breakfast

Coffee or tea (with ½ squeezed lemon)

Hazelnut milk, unsweetened (1 glass, 240 mL)

Walnut bread (60 g)

Strawberry jam, no sugar added (20 g, 1 tbsp)

Lunch

Pumpkin soup with croutons (broccoli soup may be substituted)

Pumpkin or squash, peeled, seeded, and chopped (300 g)

Olive oil (12 mL, 1 tbsp)

Chili flakes (optional)

Onion (optional)

Parsley

Salt and pepper to taste

Croutons (40 g)

Pumpkin seeds (9 g, 1 tsp)

Boil the pumpkin or squash in salted water. When cooked, drain the water. Add the oil, chili flakes, onion, parsley, and salt and pepper to taste. Stir well. When soup reaches the desired consistency, puree it with a hand blender. Serve in a bowl garnished with the croutons and pumpkin seeds.

Side dish: mixed green salad with cucumbers, carrots, and tomatoes with brown bread (40 g)

Snack

Fresh mixed-berry smoothie (150 g) and banana (1 medium); or hazelnut milk (1 glass, 240 mL) and a nut and whole-grain dark chocolate bar; choose a brand containing 150 calories, low in sugar (less than 8 g), made with 70% minimum dark chocolate and no milk

Dinner

Pasta with tuna, olives, capers, and tomato

Pasta, any type (40 g)

Tuna (60 g)

Olives (20 g)

Tomatoes (150 g) (cut in cubes/pieces)

Garlic (optional) (cut in half)

Olive oil (25 mL, 2 tbsp)

Parsley

Salt and pepper

Bring a large pot of water to boil and cook the pasta. In a separate pan, cook the tuna, olives, tomatoes, and garlic in a little water. Add the drained pasta when it's ready. Stir in the olive oil and let the mixture rest for a few minutes. Add parsley and salt and pepper to taste.

Side dish: artichokes (150 g), boiled and seasoned with oil and lemon accompanied with brown bread (40 g)

Suggested dessert: hazelnuts (25 g) and grapes (100 g), or raisins (20 g)

WEEK 2

DAY 3

Breakfast

Coffee or tea (with ½ squeezed lemon)

Cinnamon raisin bagel or 2 pieces of toast (80 g)

Plum jam, no sugar added (20 g, 1 tbsp)

Lunch

Rice with zucchini and peas

Rice (40 g)

Zucchini (250 g)

Peas (100 g)

Onion (1 medium), chopped

Olive oil (12 mL, 1 tbsp)

Parsley

Salt and pepper

Parmesan cheese (1 tbsp) or pesto (1 tsp)

Boil the rice in salted water. Drain and set it aside. In a separate pan, stir the zucchini, peas, and onion in water. Drain the vegetables, stir in parsley and salt and pepper to taste. Add the rice and olive oil and let it rest for 2 to 3 minutes. Add Parmesan or pesto, as preferred, and serve.

Snack

Coconut milk, unsweetened (1 glass, 240 mL)

Nut and whole-grain dark chocolate bar; choose a brand containing 150 calories, low in sugar (less than 8 g), made with 70% minimum dark chocolate and no milk

Dinner

White bean salad with onion, rosemary, and chicory

Chicory or other green leafy vegetable (180 g)

Gralic (1 clove cut in half)

Cherry tomatoes (50 grams).

Chili flakes to taste

Onion (1 medium)

White cannellini beans (150 g, wet, drained), cooked

Olive oil (25 mL, 2 tbsp)

Salt and pepper

Rosemary sprig

Dried whole-wheat focaccia, with olive oil (40 g)

Boil the chicory in salted water. Drain it well. Place the leaves in a pan with garlic, cherry tomatoes, onion chili flakes, and enough water to prevent drying. Cook for 5 minutes. In a separate bowl, season the cooked cannellini beans with olive oil, salt and pepper, and rosemary leaves. Combine the chicory and cannellini mixtures and serve warm or cold, as desired.

Suggested dessert: almonds (25 g) and cherries (80 g) or dried cherries (20 g)

DAY 4

Breakfast

Coffee, espresso or American

Almond milk, unsweetened (1 glass, 240 mL)

Raisin and walnut bread (60 g)

Banana (1 medium)

Lunch

Fennel salad with tomatoes, carrots, onions, and olives

Fennel bulb (150 g)

Cherry tomatoes (150 g)

Carrots (1 medium)

Onion (1 medium)

Olives (20 g)

Olive oil (12 mL, 1 tbsp)

Parsley

Salt

Whole-wheat dried focaccia, with extra virgin olive oil (40 g) (on the side)

Side dish: chicory (200 g), boiled and seasoned with oil and lemon

Side dish: mixed green salad with cucumbers, carrots, and tomatoes

Snack

Goat's milk yogurt (125 g)

Nut and whole-grain dark chocolate bar; choose a brand containing 150 calories, low in sugar (less than 8 g), made with 70% minimum dark chocolate and no milk

Dinner

Black/venus rice with zucchini and shrimp

Black/venus rice (40 g)

Zucchini (250 g) (sliced)

Cherry tomatoes (150 g)

Shrimp (60 g)

Parmesan cheese (5 g, 1 tbsp)

Saffron (4 g)

Olive oil (25 mL, 2 tbsp)

Parsley

Salt and pepper

Cook the rice following the package instructions. In a separate pan, cook the zucchini, tomatoes, and shrimp in water. Drain and mix them with the cooked rice, stirring in the Parmesan cheese, saffron, and olive oil. Season with parsley and salt and pepper to taste.

Side dish: mixed green salad with tomatoes and carrots (200 g), seasoned with balsamic vinegar

Suggested dessert: dried cranberries (20 g) and walnuts (25 g)

Take a complete multivitamin and mineral pill and one omega-3 oil soft gel.

DAY 5

Breakfast

Tea (1 black and 1 green tea bag) with 1 freshly squeezed
lemon

Whole-wheat Rice Krispies bar (60 g)

Banana (1 medium)

Dark chocolate (30 g)

Lunch

Mediterranean spelt salad with artichokes and mushrooms

Spelt (40 g)

Artichokes, preserved in oil (80 g)

Carrot (1 medium), chopped

Cherry tomatoes (150 g)

Olives (20 g)

Olive oil (12 g, 1 tbsp)

Salt and pepper

Mushrooms (150 g)

Garlic (1 clove)

Parsley

Boil the spelt in salted water until cooked. Drain and place
it in a bowl. Add the artichokes, carrot, tomatoes, and
olives. Season with oil, salt and pepper, and additional
herbs, if desired. In a separate pan, boil the mushrooms
with garlic and water. When the mushrooms are tender,
add the parsley and salt to taste. Stir in the oil. Enjoy

the mushrooms separately or add them to the rest of the ingredients.

Side dish: mixed green salad, seasoned with balsamic vinegar

Snack

Almond milk, unsweetened (1 glass, 240 mL)

Nut and whole-grain dark chocolate bar; choose a brand containing 150 calories, low in sugar (less than 8 g), made with 70% minimum dark chocolate and no milk

Dinner

Ligurian minestrone (*minestrone alla Genovese*)

Cannellini beans (150 g wet weight, drained)

Potato (1 medium)

Eggplant (1 medium)

Zucchini (1 medium)

Cabbage (1 medium)

Peas (1 handful)

Green beans (150 g)

Garlic (1 clove)

Salt and pepper

Pasta (40 g)

Olive oil (25 mL, 2 tbsp)

Pesto (1 tsp)

Boil the soaked beans in a pot of water. Chop all the vegetables in small pieces and add them to the pot, along with the garlic and salt and pepper. Cook the soup for about 45 minutes, then add the pasta. When the pasta is cooked, stir in the olive oil and pesto and remove the pot from the heat.

Side dish: mixed green salad with whole-wheat bread (40 g)

Suggested dessert: fresh fruit (e.g., 150 g of grapes)

WEEK 2

DAY 6

Breakfast

Coffee or tea

Hazelnut milk, unsweetened (1 glass, 240 mL)

Fruit and nut cereal (60 g)

Lunch

Tomato soup with basil, pesto, and croutons

Tomatoes (500 g)

Carrot (1 medium)

Celery (1 medium)

Potato (1 medium)

Red onion (1/2 medium)

Olive oil (12 g, 1 tbsp)

Basil (5 leaves)

Salt and pepper to taste

Pesto (5 g, 1 tsp)

Croutons (40 g)

Boil the tomatoes, carrot, celery, potato, and onion in a pan with salted water. When vegetables are tender, puree them with a hand blender. Add the oil, basil, and salt and pepper. Serve garnished with pesto and croutons.

Side dish: mixed green salad with carrots and tomato; or boiled green leafy vegetables (200 g) with brown bread (40 g)

Snack

Hazelnut milk, unsweetened (1 glass, 240 mL)

Nut whole-grain dark chocolate bar; choose a brand containing 150 calories, low in sugar (less than 8 g), made with 70% minimum dark chocolate and no milk

Dinner

Cream of garbanzo beans (*vellutata di ceci*) + steamed broccoli

Garbanzo beans (150 g wet weight, drained)

Rosemary (1 sprig)

Garlic (1 clove, cut in ½)

Olive oil (25 mL, 2 tbsp)

Salt and pepper to taste

Broccoli, boiled and seasoned with oil and lemon (150 g)

Garbanzo bean bread (page 228) or whole-wheat focaccia, with olive oil (60 g)

Boil the soaked garbanzo beans in salted water with the garlic and rosemary. When cooked, drain and puree with a hand blender. Add the oil and salt and pepper and let the soup rest.

Steam the broccoli until tender, then season with oil, salt, and lemon. Serve the soup and steamed broccoli with your choice of garbanzo bean bread or whole-wheat focaccia.

Suggested dessert: dried apricots (20 g) and almonds (25 g)

WEEK 2

DAY 7

Breakfast

Coffee or tea

Almond milk, unsweetened (1 glass, 240 mL)

Cranberry bread (80 g)

Honey (10 g, 2 tsp)

Lunch

Barley salad with broccoli, feta, and tomatoes

Barley (40 g)

Broccoli (150 g)

Cherry tomatoes (100 g)

Carrots (1 medium)

Onion (optional)

Feta cheese (20 g)

Olive oil (12 mL, 1 tbsp)

Parsley

Salt and pepper

Boil the barley in salted water. In a separate pan, steam the broccoli. When both are cooked, drain well and set aside to cool. Mix the barley and broccoli in a bowl and add the raw chopped cherry tomatoes, carrots, and onion. Stir in the feta cheese. Season with the oil, parsley, and salt and pepper to taste. Serve warm or cold.

Side dish: leafy green vegetables, seasoned with oil and lemon and brown bread (40 g)

Snack

Coconut milk, unsweetened (1 glass, 240 mL)

Nut and whole-grain dark chocolate bar; choose a brand containing 150 calories, low in sugar (less than 8 g), made with 70% minimum dark chocolate and no milk

Dinner

Pizza with vegetables, anchovies, and sardines (no cheese)

Pizza crust, ready-made (100 g)

Sardines and anchovies (90 g)

Cherry tomatoes (80 g)

Artichokes, canned (50 g)

Mushrooms (100 g), sliced

Spinach (100 g)

Pepper (100 g)

Olives, black (20 g)

Olive oil (25 g, 2 tbsp)

Salt and pepper to taste

Top your ready-made pizza crust with the fish, all the vegetables, and the olives. Season with oil, salt and pepper, and any herbs and spices you prefer. Bake according to the instructions on the crust package. You can also try different combinations of vegetables and fish, but remember that anchovies and sardines are rich in omega-3 fatty acids.

Suggested dessert: unsalted pistachios (25 g) and dried cranberries (20 g)

Take a complete multivitamin and mineral pill and one omega-3 oil soft gel.

Appendix B:
Food Sources of
Vitamins and Minerals

Food Sources of Vitamin B12

Food	Serving Size	Vitamin B12 Micrograms	Percent Daily Value (DV)
Tuna fish, bluefin, raw or cooked	75 g (2½ oz)	8.2–9.3	137–155
Clams, cooked	75 g (2½ oz)	74.2	1,237
Mussels, cooked	75 g (2½ oz)	25	417
Oysters, cooked	75 g (2½ oz)	18.2	303
Mackerel (king, Atlantic), cooked	75 g (2½ oz)	14	233
Roe, raw	75 g (2½ oz)	9	150
Crab, Alaska king, cooked	75 g (2½ oz)	8.6	143
Herring, cooked or kippered	250 mL (1 cup)	7.2	120
Sardines, canned in oil or tomato sauce	75 g (2½ oz)	6.8	113
Caviar (black, red)	75 g (2½ oz)	6	100
Breakfast cereal, fortified with 100% of the DV for vitamin B12	1 serving	6	100

Food	Serving Size	Vitamin B12 Micrograms	Percent Daily Value (DV)
Trout, cooked	75 g (2½ oz)	5	83
Salmon, red/sockeye, cooked	75 g (2½ oz)	4	67
Salmon, pink/humpback, with bones, canned	75 g (2½ oz)	3.7	62
Fish, tuna fish, light, canned in oil, drained solids	1.0 cup	3.21	54
Salmon, red/sockeye, cooked	75 g (2½ oz)	2.3	38
Salmon, Atlantic, wild, cooked	75 g (2½ oz)	2.3	38
Tuna fish, light, canned in water	75 g (2½ oz)	2.2	37
Soy burger	75 g (2½ oz)	1.8	30
Almond, oat, or rice milk beverage, fortified	250 mL (1 cup)	1	17
Red Star T6635+ Yeast (Vegetarian Support Formula)	2 grams	1	17
Breakfast cereals, fortified with 25% of the DV for vitamin B12	1 serving	1	17
Egg, cooked, hard-boiled	1 large	0.6	10

Sources:

https://ndb.nal.usda.gov/

http://www.fda.gov/Food/GuidanceRegulation/GuidanceDocumentsRegulatoryInformation/LabelingNutrition/ucm064928.htm

http://www.ncbi.nlm.nih.gov/pmc/articles/PMC3174857

http://www.ncbi.nlm.nih.gov/pubmed/24724766

https://www.dietitians.ca/Your-Health/Nutrition-A-Z/Vitamins/Food-Sources-of-Vitamin-B12.aspx http://www.ncbi.nlm.nih.gov/pmc/articles/PMC3174857/

http://www.ncbi.nlm.nih.gov/pubmed/24724766

Food Sources of Folate

Food	Serving Size	Micrograms per Serving	Percent Daily Value
Spinach, boiled	½ cup	131	33
Black-eyed peas (cowpeas), boiled	½ cup	105	26
Breakfast cereal, fortified with 25% of the DV for folate	1 cup	100	25
Rice, white, medium-grain, cooked	½ cup	90	23
Asparagus, boiled	4 spears	89	22
Spaghetti, enriched, cooked	½ cup	83	21
Brussels sprouts, frozen, boiled	½ cup	78	20
Lettuce, romaine, shredded	1 cup	64	16
Avocado, raw, sliced	½ cup	59	15
Spinach, raw	1 cup	58	15
Broccoli, chopped, frozen, cooked	½ cup	52	13
Mustard greens, chopped, frozen, boiled	½ cup	52	13
Green peas, frozen, boiled	½ cup	47	12
Kidney beans, canned	½ cup	46	12
Bread, white	1 slice	43	11
Peanuts, dry roasted	1 oz	41	10
Wheat germ	2 tbsp	40	10
Tomato juice, canned	¾ cup	36	9
Crab, Dungeness	3 oz	36	9
Orange juice	¾ cup	35	9
Turnip greens, frozen, boiled	½ cup	32	8
Orange, fresh	1 small	29	7
Papaya, raw, cubed	½ cup	27	7

Food	Serving Size	Micrograms per Serving	Percent Daily Value
Banana	1 medium	24	6
Yeast, baker's	¼ tsp	23	6
Egg, hard-boiled	1 large	22	6
Cantaloupe, raw	1 wedge	14	4
Halibut, cooked	3 oz	12	3

Food Sources of Calcium

Food	Serving Size	Milligrams per Serving	Percent Daily Value
Breakfast cereal, fortified with calcium	1 cup	100–1,000	10–100
Beverages, coconut milk, sweetened, fortified with calcium and vitamins A, B12, and D2	1 cup	451	45
Beverages, chocolate almond milk, unsweetened, shelf-stable, fortified with vitamins D2 and E	1 cup	451	45
Beverages, vanilla almond milk, sweetened	8 fl oz	451	45
Almonds, whole	1 cup	385	39
Chickpeas (garbanzo beans, bengal gram), mature seeds, canned, drained	1 cup	370	37
Soy milk (all flavors), enhanced	1 cup	340	34
Sardines, canned in oil, with bones	3 oz	325	33
Soy milk, fortified with calcium	8 oz	299	30
Collards, cooked, boiled, drained, without salt	1 cup	268	27

Food	Serving Size	Milligrams per Serving	Percent Daily Value
Orange juice, fortified with calcium	6 oz	261	26
Salmon, pink, canned, solids with bone	3 oz	181	18
Seeds, chia seeds, dried	1 oz	179	18
Salmon, red/sockeye, canned	3 oz	168	17
Beet greens, cooked, boiled, drained, without salt	1 cup (1-inch pieces)	164	16
Crustaceans, lobster, northern, cooked with moist heat	1 cup	139	14
Hazelnuts or filberts	1 cup	131	13
Peanuts, Virginia, raw	1 cup	130	13
Pistachios, raw	1 cup	129	13
Trout, rainbow, wild, cooked, dry heat	1 fillet	123	12
Black turtle beans, mature seeds, cooked, boiled, without salt	1 cup	102	10
Kale, raw, chopped	1 cup	100	10
Turnip greens, fresh, boiled	½ cup	99	10
Kale, fresh, cooked	1 cup	94	9
Squash, winter, acorn, cooked, baked, without salt	1 cup	90	9
White beans, cooked	½ cup	81	8
Chinese cabbage, bok choy, raw, shredded	1 cup	74	7
Bread, white	1 slice	73	7
Anchovies, European, canned in oil, drained solids, boneless	1 oz	66	7
Salmon, red/sockeye, fillets with skin, smoked (Alaska Native)	1 fillet	63	6

Food	Serving Size	Milligrams per Serving	Percent Daily Value
Sweet potato, baked, with salt	1 cup	62	6
Figs, dried	¼ cup	61	6
Tortilla, corn, ready-to-bake/fry	6-in diameter	46	5
Pinto beans, cooked	½ cup	39	4
Tortilla, flour, ready-to-bake/fry	6-in diameter	32	3
Bread, whole wheat	1 slice	30	3
Red beans, cooked	½ cup	25	3
Broccoli, raw	½ cup	21	2

The DV for calcium is 1,000 milligrams for adults and children ages four years and older.
Source: https://ods.od.nih.gov/factsheets/Calcium-HealthProfessional

Food Sources of Iron

Food	Serving Size	Milligrams per Serving	Percent Daily Value
Seaweed, spirulina, dried	1 cup	31.92	177
Breakfast cereal, fortified with 100% of the DV for iron	1 serving	18	100
Cocoa, dry powder, unsweetened	1 cup	12	67
Oysters, eastern, cooked with moist heat	3 oz	8	44
White beans, canned	1 cup	8	44
Chocolate, dark, 45%–69% cacao solids	3 oz	7	39
Mollusks, mussels, blue, cooked, moist heat	3 oz	5.71	32
Peanut butter, chunky, vitamin and mineral fortified	2 tbsp	5.6	31

Food	Serving Size	Milligrams per Serving	Percent Daily Value
Almonds, whole	1 cup	5.31	30
Mixed nuts, dry roasted, with peanuts, without salt added	1 cup	4.89	27
Lentils, boiled and drained	½ cup	3	17
Spinach, boiled and drained	½ cup	3	17
Kidney beans, canned	½ cup	2	11
Sardines, Atlantic, canned in oil, drained solids with bone	3 oz	2	11
Chickpeas (garbanzo beans, bengal gram), boiled and drained	½ cup	2	11
Tomatoes, stewed, canned	½ cup	2	11
Potato, baked, flesh and skin	1 medium	2	11
Cashew nuts, oil roasted	1 oz (18 nuts)	2	11
Green peas, boiled	½ cup	1	6
Rice, white, long grain, enriched, parboiled, drained	½ cup	1	6
Bread, whole wheat	1 slice	1	6
Bread, white	1 slice	1	6
Raisins, seedless	¼ cup	1	6
Spaghetti, whole wheat, cooked	1 cup	1	6
Tuna, bluefin, fresh, cooked with dry heat	3 oz	1	6
Pistachios, dry roasted	1 oz (49 nuts)	1	6
Broccoli, boiled and drained	½ cup	1	6
Egg, hard-boiled	1 large	1	6
Rice, brown, long, or medium grain, cooked	1 cup	1	6

Source: https://ods.od.nih.gov/factsheets/Iron-HealthProfessional

Food Sources of Vitamin A

Food	Serving Size	Micrograms of Retinol Activity Equivalents (RAE) per Serving	International Units (IU) per Serving	Percent Daily Value
Sweet potato, baked in skin	1 whole	1,403	28,058	561
Spinach, frozen, boiled	½ cup	573	11,458	229
Carrots, raw	½ cup	459	9,189	184
Pumpkin pie, commercially prepared	1 piece	488	3,743	75
Cantaloupe, raw	½ cup	135	2,706	54
Peppers, sweet, red, raw	½ cup	117	2,332	47
Mangos, raw	1 whole	112	2,240	45
Black-eyed peas (cowpeas), boiled	1 cup	66	1,305	26
Apricots, dried, sulfured	10 halves	63	1,261	25
Broccoli, boiled	½ cup	60	1,208	24
Tomato juice, canned	¾ cup	42	821	16
Herring, Atlantic, pickled	3 oz	219	731	15
Breakfast cereal, fortified with 10% of the DV for vitamin A	¾–1 cup	127–149	500	10
Baked beans, canned, plain or vegetarian	1 cup	13	274	5
Egg, hard-boiled	1 large	75	260	5
Summer squash, all varieties, boiled	½ cup	10	191	4
Salmon, red/sockeye, cooked	3 oz	59	176	4
Yogurt, plain, low fat	1 cup	32	116	2
Pistachio nuts, dry roasted	1 oz	4	73	1
Tuna, light, canned in oil, drained solids	3 oz	20	65	1

Food Sources of Vitamin C

Food	Serving Size	Milligrams per Serving	Percent Daily Value
Red pepper, sweet, raw	½ cup	95	158
Orange juice	¾ cup	93	155
Orange	1 medium	70	117
Grapefruit juice	¾ cup	70	117
Kiwifruit	1 medium	64	107
Green pepper, sweet, raw	½ cup	60	100
Broccoli, cooked	½ cup	51	85
Strawberries, fresh, sliced	½ cup	49	82
Brussels sprouts, cooked	½ cup	48	80
Grapefruit juice	½ medium	39	65
Broccoli, raw	½ cup	39	65
Tomato juice	¾ cup	33	55
Cantaloupe	½ cup	29	48
Cabbage, cooked	½ cup	28	47
Cauliflower, raw	½ cup	26	43
Potato, baked	1 medium	17	28
Tomato, raw	1 medium	17	28
Spinach, cooked	½ cup	9	15
Green peas, frozen, cooked	½ cup	8	13

Food Sources of Vitamin D

Food	Serving Size	International Units (IU) per Serving	Percent Daily Value
Cod liver oil	1 tbsp	1,360	340
Maitake mushrooms, raw	1 cup	786	196.5
Swordfish, cooked	3 oz	566	141.5
Trout, rainbow, farmed, cooked, dry heat	1 fillet	539	134.75
Salmon, red/sockeye, cooked	3 oz	447	111.75
Herring, Atlantic, cooked, dry heat	1 fillet	306	76.5
Tuna, canned in water, drained	3 oz	154	38.5
Tilapia, raw	1 fillet	144	36
Orange juice, fortified with vitamin D	1 cup	137	34.25
Soymilk (all flavors), enhanced	1 cup	114	28.5
Chanterelle mushrooms, raw	1 cup	114	28.5
Beverages, almond milk, chocolate	8 fl oz	101	25.25
Beverages, coconut milk, sweetened, fortified with calcium and vitamins A, B12, and D2	1 cup	101	25.25
Beverages, rice milk, unsweetened	8 fl oz	101	25.25
Sardines, canned in oil, drained	2 sardines	46	11.5
Salmon, Atlantic, farmed, cooked, dry heat	3 oz	44	11
Egg (vitamin D is found in the yolk)	1 large	41	10.25
Shiitake mushrooms, cooked without salt	1 cup	41	10.25

Food	Serving Size	International Units (IU) per Serving	Percent Daily Value
Breakfast cereal, fortified with 10% of the DV for vitamin D	¾–1 cup	40	10
Anchovy, European, canned in oil, drained solids, boneless	1 oz	20	5
White mushrooms, cooked, boiled, drained, without salt	1 cup	12	3

Selected Food Sources of Vitamin E (Alpha-Tocopherol)

Food	Serving Size	Milligrams per Serving	Percent Daily Value
Wheat germ oil	1 tbsp	20.3	102
Sunflower seeds, dry roasted	1 oz	7.4	37
Almonds, dry roasted	1 oz	6.8	34
Sunflower oil	1 tbsp	5.6	28
Safflower oil	1 tbsp	4.6	23
Hazelnuts, dry roasted	1 oz	4.3	22
Peanut butter	2 tbsp	2.9	15
Peanuts, dry roasted	1 oz	2.2	11
Corn oil	1 tbsp	1.9	10
Spinach, boiled	½ cup	1.9	10
Broccoli, chopped, boiled	½ cup	1.2	6
Soybean oil	1 tbsp	1.1	6
Kiwifruit	1 medium	1.1	6
Mango, sliced	½ cup	0.7	4
Tomato, raw	1 medium	0.7	4
Spinach, raw	1 cup	0.6	3

Food Sources of Omega-3

Food	Serving Size	Alpha-linolenic Acid (ALA) (g)	Eicosapentaenoic (EPA) / Docosahexaenoic (DHA) (g)
Halibut, cooked	75 g (2½ oz)	0.04–0.06	0.35–0.88
Herring, cooked	75 g (2½ oz)	0.05–0.11	1.6
Lobster, cooked	75 g (2½ oz)	0.01	0.42
Mackerel, cooked	75 g (2½ oz)	0.03–0.08	0.90–1.39
Mackerel, salted	75 g (2½ oz)	0.12	3.43
Mussels, cooked	75 g (2½ oz)	0.03	0.59
Octopus, cooked	75 g (2½ oz)	0	0.13
Oysters, Eastern/Blue Point, cooked	75 g (2½ oz)	0.04–0.05	0.33–0.41
Oysters, Pacific, cooked	75 g (2½ oz)	0.05	1.04
Pollock, cooked	75 g (2½ oz)	0	0.4
Salmon, Atlantic, farmed, raw or cooked	75 g (2½ oz)	0.08–0.11	1.48–1.61
Salmon, Atlantic, wild, raw or cooked	75 g (2½ oz)	0.22–0.28	1.08–1.38
Salmon, Chinook, raw or cooked	75 g (2½ oz)	0.06–0.08	1.31–1.47
Salmon, coho, raw or cooked	75 g (2½ oz)	0.03–0.05	0.33–0.98
Salmon, pink/humpback, raw, cooked or canned	75 g (2½ oz)	0.03–0.06	0.96–1.26
Salmon, red/sockeye, raw, cooked or canned	75 g (2½ oz)	0.05–0.07	0.87–1.06
Sardines, canned	75 g (2½ oz)	0.17–0.37	0.74–1.05
Scallops, cooked	75 g (2½ oz)	0	0.27
Shrimp, cooked	75 g (2½ oz)	0.01	0.24
Snapper, cooked	75 g (2½ oz)	0	0.25
Sole or plaice, cooked	75 g (2½ oz)	0.01	0.37
Tilapia, cooked	75 g (2½ oz)	0.03	0.1

Food	Serving Size	Alpha-linolenic Acid (ALA) (g)	Eicosapentaenoic (EPA) / Docosahexaenoic (DHA) (g)
Trout, cooked	75 g (2½ oz)	0.06–0.14	0.65–0.87
Tuna, light, canned with water	75 g (2½ oz)	0	0.21
Tuna, white, canned with water	75 g (2½ oz)	0.05	0.65
Whitefish, cooked	75 g (2½ oz)	0.17	1.2
Beans (navy, pinto), cooked	175 mL (¾ cup)	0.17–0.24	0
Peas, black-eyed, cooked	175 mL (¾ cup)	0.11	0
Soybeans, mature, cooked	175 mL (¾ cup)	0.76	0
Meatless fish sticks, chicken, or meatballs, cooked	75 g (2½ oz)	0.39–0.78	0
Almonds, oil roasted, blanched	60 mL (¼ cup)	0.15	0
Chia seeds	15 mL (1 tbsp)	1.9	0
Flaxseed, ground*	15 mL (1 tbsp)	2.46	0
Hickory nuts	60 mL (¼ cup)	0.32	0
Pumpkin seeds, without shell	60 mL (¼ cup)	0.06	0
Pecans	60 mL (¼ cup)	0.25–0.29	0
Soy nuts	60 mL (¼ cup)	0.42	0
Walnuts, black	60 mL (¼ cup	0.64	0
Walnuts, English, Persian	60 mL (¼ cup)	2.3	0
Canola oil	5 mL (1 tsp)	0.42	0
DHA-enriched omega-3 margarine made with fish oil	5 mL (1 tsp)	0.28	0.03
Flaxseed oil	5 mL (1 tsp)	2.58	0
Omega-3 margarine made with canola oil*	5 mL (1 tsp)	0.34	0
Soybean oil	5 mL (1 tsp)	0.31	0
Walnut oil	5 mL (1 tsp)	0.48	0
Herring oil supplement	5 mL (1 tsp)	0.04	0.48

Food	Serving Size	Alpha-linolenic Acid (ALA) (g)	Eicosapentaenoic (EPA) / Docosahexaenoic (DHA) (g)
Salmon oil supplement	5 mL (1 tsp)	0.05	1.44
Sardine oil supplement	5 mL (1 tsp)	0.06	0.96
Almond milk beverage	250 mL (1 cup)	0.1	0
Oat beverage	250 mL (1 cup)	0.3	0

* Amounts vary depending on the product.

Source: http://www.whfoods.com/genpage.php?dbid=84&tname=nutrient

http://www.dietitians.ca/Your-Health/Nutrition-A-Z/Fat/Food-Sources-of
-Omega-3-Fats.aspx

Food Sources of Magnesium

Food	Serving Size	Milligrams per Serving	Percent Daily Value
Almonds, dry roasted	1 oz	80	20
Spinach, boiled	½ cup	78	20
Cashews, dry roasted	1 oz	74	19
Peanuts, oil roasted	¼ cup	63	16
Cereal, shredded wheat	2 large biscuits	61	15
Soymilk, plain or vanilla	1 cup	61	15
Black beans, cooked	½ cup	60	15
Edamame, shelled, cooked	½ cup	50	13
Peanut butter, smooth	2 tbsp	49	12
Bread, whole wheat	2 slices	46	12
Avocado, cubed	1 cup	44	11
Potato, baked with skin	3.5 oz	43	11
Rice, brown, cooked	½ cup	42	11
Breakfast cereal, fortified with 10% of the DV for magnesium	1/3 cup	40	10

Food	Serving Size	Milligrams per Serving	Percent Daily Value
Oatmeal, instant	1 packet	36	9
Kidney beans, canned	½ cup	35	9
Banana	1 medium	32	8
Salmon, Atlantic, farmed, cooked	3 oz	26	7
Halibut, cooked	3 oz	24	6
Raisins	½ cup	23	6
Broccoli, chopped and cooked	½ cup	12	3
Rice, white, cooked	½ cup	10	3
Apple	1 medium	9	2
Carrot, raw	1 medium	7	2

Source: https://ods.od.nih.gov/factsheets/Magnesium-HealthProfessional/

Acknowledgments

THIS BOOK SUMS UP THIRTY YEARS of my journey in search of the secrets of longevity, during which I was accompanied by great pioneers, and also by young and very good researchers. I thank Professor Scott Norton and Robert Gracy in Texas for giving me the opportunity to learn biochemistry and begin my studies in the aging field. I thank Professor Roy Walford of UCLA for teaching me to challenge the rules and think about aging in an innovative way. I thank Professor Joan Valentine and Edith Gralla at UCLA for giving me the solid genetic and molecular basis on which I have built my research. I thank Professor Caleb Finch at USC for introducing me to neurobiology and theories of aging, and for being a great mentor from the time I finished my doctoral studies to the present. I thank Professor Pinchas Cohen for a long series of fruitful collaborations, and for his support as Dean of the School of Gerontology at USC. I thank Professor Marco

Foiani, the director of the IFOM Institute, for giving me the opportunity to lead an oncology research group in Italy. I thank a group of pioneer geneticists for twenty-five years of endless arguments, discussions, and discoveries that have enabled us all to contribute to an extraordinary revolution in the field of aging and longevity. I am infinitely grateful to my students, researchers, and medical colleagues, without whom I would only have discovered a small fraction of what we have discovered together. Special thanks to Dr. Paola Fabrizio for her essential role in my USC laboratory findings shortly after my appointment, and Professor Min Wei for many years of leadership in the lab.

I thank all the colleagues who offered me valuable expertise from their specialized fields:

For his advice on chapter 7 I thank Professor Alessio Nencioni, a specialist of internal medicine at the Hospital San Martino, University of Genoa. Professor Nencioni is responsible for the study funded by the Umberto Foundation Veronesi on the fasting-mimicking diet and chemotherapy in breast cancer patients.

Tanya Dorff, oncologist and associate professor of clinical medicine, USC Norris Cancer Hospital, who is in charge of clinical trials on the fasting-mimicking diet and chemotherapy at USC, and Alessandro Laviano, professor of clinical medicine, University La Sapienza, Rome.

For valuable help with chapter 8 I thank Professor Hanno Pijl, endocrinologist and diabetologist, director of the Endocrinology and Metabolic Diseases Clinic of Leiden University, Holland, and Clayton Frenzel, a leading bariatric surgeon at Texas Health Harris Methodist Hospital.

Professor Andreas Michalsen, chief of complementary medicine in the Department of Integrative Medicine at the Hospital Charité in Berlin, who advised me for chapter 9. Dr. Michalsen is one of the leading experts on clinical aspects of fasting therapies, and has directed clinical trials on fasting or fasting diets and risk factors for cardiovascular disease.

Kurt Hong, MD, PhD, associate professor and director of the USC Center for Clinical Nutrition, Los Angeles. An MD/PhD from Harvard Medical School and former clinician at the UCLA Center for Human Nutrition, Dr. Hong is a leading expert in the field of clinical nutrition.

For chapter 10 I thank Dr. Markus Bock, a neurologist who is experienced in the use of ketogenic diets and fasting-mimicking diets at the Complementary Medical Center of the Charité Hospital in Berlin. Dr. Bock has conducted clinical trials on the fasting-mimicking diet and neurodegenerative diseases in collaboration with Dr. Michalsen.

Thank you to Patrizio Odetti, chief of geriatrics at the University of Genova San Martino Hospital, one of the leading geriatric programs in Italy with a large number of dementia patients.

For chapter 11 I also thank Dr. Markus Bock, Professor Andreas Michalsen, and Professor Kurt Hong, MD, PhD.

Finally, the Two-Week Meal Plan was written with the help of nutritionist Noemi Renzetti and dietitians Mahshid Shelechi and Susan Kim, to whom I owe all my gratitude.

I thank Diane Krieger and Emily H. Jackson for the initial editing of the English version of the book.

A special thank-you to Claudia Herr, for extensive editing of the English text and valuable advice.

I thank Laurie Liss at Sterling Lord Literistic for her wisdom and guidance.

I thank the whole Avery Books team at Penguin Random House: publisher Megan Newman; her assistant, Hannah Steigmeyer; Justin Thrift; Andrea Ho; and Lindsay Gordon.

Notes

CHAPTER 1

1 V.D. Longo et al., "Enhancing Stem Cell Transplantation with 'Nutri-technology,'" *Cell Stem Cell* 19, no. 6 (December 1, 2016): 681–682.

CHAPTER 2

1 V.D. Longo, J. Mitteldorf, and V.P. Skulachev, "Programmed and Altruistic Aging," *Nature Reviews Genetics* 6 (November 2005): 866–872.

2 V.D. Longo, "Mutations in Signal Transduction Proteins Increase Stress Resistance and Longevity in Yeast, Nematodes, Fruit Flies, and Mammalian Neuronal Cells," *Neurobiology of Aging* 20 (1999): 479–486; PMID: 10638521.

3 P. Fabrizio, F. Pozza, S.D. Pletcher, C.M. Gendron, and V.D. Longo, "Regulation of Longevity and Stress Resistance by Sch9 in Yeast," *Science* 292 (2001): 288–290.

4 Jaime Guevara-Aguirre, Priya Balasubramaniam, Marco Guevara-

Aguirre, et al., "Growth Hormone Receptor Deficiency Is Associated with a Major Reduction in Pro-Aging Signaling, Cancer, and Diabetes in Humans," *Science Translational Medicine* 3, no. 70 (February 16, 2011): 70ra13. http://stm.sciencemag.org/content/3/70/70ra13.full.

5 Ibid.

6 Kaoru Nashiro, Jaime Guevara-Aguirre, Meredith N. Braskie, et al., "Brain Structure and Function Associated with Younger Adults in Growth Hormone Receptor-Deficient Humans," *Journal of Neuroscience* 37, no. 7 (February 15, 2017): 1696–1707. http://www.jneurosci.org/content/37/7/1696.

7 Edward O. List et al., "Endocrine Parameters and Phenotypes of the Growth Hormone Receptor Gene Disrupted (GHR–/–) Mouse," *Endocrine Reviews* 32, no. 3 (June 2011): 356–386. http://europepmc.org/articles/PMC3365798.

CHAPTER 3

1 L. Fontana, B.K. Kennedy, and V.D. Longo, "Medical Research: Treat Ageing," *Nature* (July 24, 2014), 511(7510): 405-7, PMID: 25056047.

CHAPTER 4

1 Kaye Foster-Powell, Susanna H.A. Holt, and Janette C. Brand-Miller, "International Table of Glycemic Index and Glycemic Load Values: 2002," *American Journal of Clinicial Nutrition* (January 2002), 76: 5–56. http://ajcn.nutrition.org/content/76/1/5.full.pdf.

2 B. Frei, B.N. Ames, J.B. Blumberg, and W.C. Willett, "Enough Is Enough," *Annals of Internal Medicine* 160, no. 11 (June 3, 2014): 807.

3 "Effects of Multivitamin Supplement on Cataract and Age-Related Macular Degeneration in a Randomized Trial of Male Physicians," *Ophthalmology* (February 2014): 73, 525–534.

4 D. Belsky, A. Caspi, et al., "Quantification of Biological Aging in Young Adults," *PNAS* 112, no. 30 (July 2015).

5   L. Fontana, L. Partridge, and V.D. Longo, "Extending Healthy Life Span—from Yeast to Humans," *Science* 328, no. 5976 (April 16, 2010): 321–326.

6   S. Gill and S. Panda, "A Smartphone App Reveals Erratic Diurnal Eating Patterns in Humans That Can Be Modulated for Health Benefits," *Cell Metabolism* (November 3, 2015), 22(5): 789–98.

7   Fontana, Partridge, and Longo, "Extending Healthy Life Span."

8   S.M. Solon-Biet, "The Ratio of Macronutrients, Not Caloric Intake, Dictates Cardiometabolic Health, Aging, and Longevity in Ad Libitum-Fed Mice," *Cell Metabolism* (March 4, 2014), 19(3): 418–430.

9   M. Levine et al. and V.D. Longo, "Low Protein Intake Is Associated with a Major Reduction in IGF-1, Cancer, and Overall Mortality in the 65 and Younger but Not Older Population," *Cell Metabolism* (March 4, 2014), 19(3): 407–17.

10 S. Brandhorst et al. and V.D. Longo, "A Periodic Diet That Mimics Fasting Promotes Multi-System Regeneration, Enhanced Cognitive Performance, and Healthspan," *Cell Metabolism* (July 2015), 22(1): 86–99.

11 S. Di Biase, H.S. Shim, K.H. Kim, M. Vinciguerra, F. Rappa, M. Wei, et al., "Fasting Regulates EGR1 and Protects from Glucose- and Dexamethasone-Dependent Sensitization to Chemotherapy," *PLoS Biology* 2017 15(3): e2001951.

12 Levine et al. and Longo, "Low Protein Intake."

13 T.T. Fung, R.M. van Dam, S.E. Hankinson, M. Stampfer, W.C. Willett, and F.B. Hu, "Low-Carbohydrate Diets and All-Cause and Cause-Specific Mortality: Two Cohort Studies," *Annals of Internal Medicine* (September 7, 2010), 153(5): 289–98.

14 M. Song, T.T. Fung, F.B. Hu, W.C. Willett, V.D. Longo, A.T. Chan, E.L. Giovannucci, "Association of Animal and Plant Protein Intake With All-Cause and Cause-Specific Mortality," *JAMA Internal Medicine* (2016) 176(10): 1453–1463.

15 L. de Koning et al., "Low-Carbohydrate Diet Scores and Risk of Type 2 Diabetes in Men," *American Journal of Clinical Nutrition* (April 2011), 93(4): 844–850.

16 M. Pollack, "Insulin and Insulin-Like Growth Factor Signaling in Neoplasia," *Nature Reviews Cancer* (December 2008), 8(12): 915–28.

17 S. Wang, "Epidemiology of Vitamin D in Health and Disease," *Nutrition Research Reviews* 22 (December 2009) 25(11): 1483–1489.

18 R. Estruch et al., "Primary Prevention of Cardiovascular Disease with a Mediterranean Diet," *New England Journal of Medicine* (April 2013) 368: 1279–1290

19 Y. Bao, J. Han, F.B. Hu, E.L. Giovannucci, M.J. Stampfer, W.C. Willett, and C.S. Fuchs, "Association of Nut Consumption with Total and Cause-Specific Mortality," *New England Journal of Medicine* (November 2013) 369(21): 2001–11.

20 Gill and Panda, "A Smartphone App Reveals Erratic Diurnal Eating Patterns."

21 M.U. Yang and T.B. Van Itallie, "Composition of Weight Lost During Short-Term Weight Reduction: Metabolic Responses of Obese Subjects to Starvation and Low-Calorie Ketogenic and Nonketogenic Diets," *Journal of Clinical Investigation* (September 1976) 58(3): 722–730.

22 Levine et al. and Longo, "Low Protein Intake."

23 Elisabetta Polovedo, "Raw Eggs and No Husband Since '38 Keep Her Young at 115," *New York Times* (February 15, 2015) p. A4.

24 A. Dutta et al., "Longer Lived Parents: Protective Associations with Cancer Incidence and Overall Mortality," *Journals of Gerontology Series A: Biological Sciences and Medical Sciences* (November 2013), 68(11): 1409–1418.

25 Ibid.

CHAPTER 5

1 Paul Bowes, "Loma Linda: The Secret to a Long Healthy Life?" *BBC Magazine* (December 8, 2014).

2 D. Buettner, *The Blue Zones: 9 Lessons for Living Longer from the People Who've Lived the Longest*, 2nd ed. (Washington, DC: National Geographic Society, 2012).

3 E.F. Chackravarty, "Long Distance Running and Knee Osteoar-

thritis: A Prospective Study," *American Journal of Preventive Medicine* 35, no. 2 (August 2008): 133–138.

4 P.T. Williams, "Effects of Running and Walking on Osteoarthritis and Hip Replacement Risk," *Medicine and Science in Sports and Exercise* (July 2013), 45(7): 1292–7.

5 K. Gebel, D. Ding, T. Chey, E. Stamatakis, W.J. Brown, and A.E. Bauman, "Effect of Moderate to Vigorous Physical Activity on All-Cause Mortality in Middle-Aged and Older Australians," *JAMA Internal Medicine* 175, no. 6 (June 6, 2015): 970977, DOI: 10.1001/jamainternmed.2015.0541.

6 H. Arem et al., "Leisure Time Physical Activity and Mortality: A Detailed Pooled Analysis of the Dose-Response Relationship," *JAMA Internal Medicine* (June 2015) 175(6): 959–67.

7 D. Paddon-Jones, B.B. Rasmussen, "Dietary Protein Recommendations and the Prevention of Sarcopenia," *Current Opinion in Clinical Nutrition and Metabolic Care* (January 2009), 12(1): 86–90.

8 V. Kumar, A. Selby, D. Rankin, et al., "Age-Related Differences in the Dose-Response Relationship of Muscle Protein Synthesis to Resistance Exercise in Young and Old Men," *Journal of Physiology* (January 15, 2009) 587(1): 211–7.

CHAPTER 6

1 C-W Cheng et al., "Prolonged Fasting Reduces IGF-1/PKA to Promote Hematopoietic-Stem-Cell-Based Regeneration and Reverse Immunosuppression," *Cell Stem Cell* (June 2014), 14(6): 810–823.

2 K.K. Ray, S.R. Seshasai, S. Erqou, P. Sever, J.W. Jukema, I. Ford, and N. Sattar, "Statins and All-Cause Mortality in High-Risk Primary Prevention: A Meta-Analysis of 11 Randomized Controlled Trials Involving 65,229 Participants," *Archives of Internal Medicine* (June 2010), 170(12): 1024–31.

3 C-W Cheng, V. Villani, R. Buono, M. Wei, S. Kumar, P. Cohen, J.B. Sneddon, L. Perin, and V.D. Longo, "Fasting-Mimicking Diet Induces Pancreatic Lineage Reprogramming to Promote Ngn3-Driven β-cell Regeneration," *Cell* 168, no. 5 (February 2017): 1–14.

CHAPTER 7

1 Yandong Shi, Emanuela Felley-Bosco, Thomas M. Marti, Katrin Orlowski, Martin Pruschy, Rolf A. Stahel, "Starvation-Induced Activation of ATM/Chk2/p53 Signaling Sensitizes Cancer Cells to Cisplatin," *BMC Cancer* 12, no. 1 (2012): 571.

2 Stefano Di Biase et al., "Fasting-Mimicking Diet Reduces HO-1 to Promote T Cell-Mediated Tumor Cytotoxicity," *Cancer Cell* 30, no. 1 (July 11, 2016): 136–146. PMC. Web. July 9, 2017. http://pubmed centralcanada.ca/pmcc/articles/PMC5388544/]

3 Ibid.

4 S. Di Biase, H.S. Shim, K.H. Kim, M. Vinciguerra, F. Rappa, M. Wei, et al., "Fasting Regulates EGR1 and Protects from Glucose- and Dexamethasone-Dependent Sensitization to Chemotherapy," *PLoS Biology* 15, no. 5 (2017): e1002603. https://doi.org/10.1371/journal.pbio.1002603.

5 M.A. Weiser, M.E. Cabanillas, M. Konopleva, D.A. Thomas, S.A. Pierce, C.P. Escalante, et al., "Relation Between the Duration of Remission and Hyperglycemia During Induction Chemotherapy for Acute Lymphocytic Leukemia with a Hyperfractionated Cyclophosphamide, Vincristine, Doxorubicin, and Dexamethasone/Methotrexate-Cytarabine Regimen," *Cancer* 100, no. 6 (March 15, 2004): 1179–1185.

6 T.B. Dorff et al., "Safety and Feasibility of Fasting in Combination with Platinum-Based Chemotherapy," *BMC Cancer* (June 2016) 16: 360.

7 S. De Groot et al., "The Effects of Short-Term Fasting on Tolerance to (Neo) Adjuvant Chemotherapy in HER2-Negative Breast Cancer Patients: A Randomized Pilot Study," *BMC Cancer* (October 2015) 15: 652.

CHAPTER 8

1 W.C. Willett, W.H. Dietz, G.A. Colditz, "Guidelines for Healthy Weight," *New England Journal of Medicine* (August 1999) 341: 427–434.

2 T. Pischon, H. Boeing, K. Hoffmann, et al., "General and Abdominal Adiposity and Risk of Death in Europe," *New England Journal of Medicine* (November 13, 2008) 359: 2105–2120.

3 R.J Colman, T.M. Beasley, J.W. Kemnitz, S.T. Johnson, R. Weindruch, and R.M. Anderson, "Caloric Restriction Reduces Age-Related and All-Cause Mortality in Rhesus Monkeys," *Nature Communications* (April 1, 2014), 5: 3557; R.L. Walford, D. Mock, R. Verdery, and T. MacCallum, "Calorie Restriction in Biosphere 2: Alterations in Physiologic, Hematologic, Hormonal, and Biochemical Parameters in Humans Restricted for a 2-Year Period," *Journals of Gerontology* (June 2002), 57(6): B211–24.

4 A.R. Barnosky, K.K. Hoody, T.G. Unterman, and K.A. Varady, "Intermittent Fasting vs. Daily Calorie Restriction for Type 2 Diabetes Prevention: A Review of Human Findings," *Translation Research* (October 2014), 164(4): 302–11.

5 S. Gill and S. Panda, "A Smartphone App Reveals Erratic Diurnal Eating Patterns in Humans That Can Be Modulated for Health Benefits," *Cell Metabolism* (November 3, 2015), 22(5): 789–98.

6 Marie-Pierre St-Onge, Jamy Ard, Monica L. Baskin, Stephanie E. Chiuve, Heather M. Johnson, Penny Kris-Etherton, and Krista Varady, "Meal Timing and Frequency: Implications for Cardiovascular Disease Prevention: A Scientific Statement from the American Heart Association," *Circulation* 135 (January 30, 2017). https://doi.org/10.1161/CIR.0000000000000476.

7 L. de Koning et al., "Low-Carbohydrate Diet Scores and Risk of Type 2 Diabetes in Men," *American Journal of Clinical Nutrition* 93, no. 4 (April 2011).

8 Levine et al. and V.D. Longo, "Low Protein Intake."

9 J. Guevara-Aguirre, A.L. Rosenbloom, P. Balasubramanian, E. Teran, M. Guevara-Aguirre, C. Guevara, P. Procel, I. Alfaras, R. De Cabo, S. Di Biase, L. Narvaez, J. Saavedra, and V.D. Longo, "GH Receptor Deficiency in Ecuadorian Adults Is Associated with Obesity and Enhanced Insulin Sensitivity," *Journal of Clinical Endocrinology and Metabolism* (July 2015), 100(7): 2589–96.

10 M.N. Harvie et al., "The Effects of Intermittent or Continuous Energy Restriction on Weight Loss and Metabolic Disease Risk Markers: A Randomized Trial in Young Overweight Women," *International Journal of Obesity* (May 2011) 35(5): 714–27.

11 Barnosky, Hoody, Unterman, and Varady, "Intermittent Fasting vs. Daily Calorie Restriction."

12 C-W Cheng et al., "Fasting-Mimicking Diet Promotes Ngn3-Driven β-Cell Regeneration to Reverse Diabetes," *Cell* (February 2017), 168(5): 775–788.e12.

13 Sripal Bangalore, Rana Fayyad, Rachel Laskey, David A. DeMicco, Franz H. Messerli, and David D. Waters, "Body Weight Outcomes in Coronary Disease," *New England Journal of Medicine* 376 (April 6, 2017): 1332–1340, DOI: 10.1056/NEJMoa1606148; K.D. Hall, "Diet Versus Exercise in 'The Biggest Loser' Weight Loss Competition," *Obesity* 21: 957–959, DOI: 10.1002/oby.20065.

CHAPTER 9

1 R.J. Colman, R.M. Anderson, et al., "Caloric Restriction Delays Disease Onset and Mortality in Rhesus Monkeys," *Science* 325, no. 5937 (July 10, 2009); R.J. Colman, T.M. Beasley, et al., "Caloric Restriction Reduces Age-Related and All-Cause Mortality in Rhesus Monkeys," *Nature* (April 2014), 325(5937): 201–4.

2 Colman, Anderson, et al., "Caloric Restriction Delays Disease Onset."

3 J.A. Mattison, G.S. Roth, et al., "Impact of Caloric Restriction on Health and Survival in Rhesus Monkeys from the NIA Study," *Nature* (September 2012), 489(7415): 318–21.

4 F. Sofi, F. Cesari, et al., "Adherence to Mediterranean Diet and Health Status: Meta-Analysis," *British Medical Journal* (September 2008); M.A. Martinez-Gonzalez, M. Bes-Rastrollo, et al., "Mediterranean Food Pattern and the Primary Prevention of Chronic Disease: Recent Developments," *Nutrition Reviews* (May 2009), 6(9): 3474–3500; F. Sofi, R. Abbate, et al., "Accruing Evidence on Benefits of Adherence to the Mediterranean Diet on Health: An

Updated Systematic Review and Meta-Analysis," *American Journal of Clinical Nutrition* (November 2010), 92(5): 1189–96.

5 F. Sofi, C. Macchi, et al., "Mediterranean Diet and Health Status: An Updated Meta-Analysis and a Proposal for a Literature-Based Adherence Score," *Public Health Nutrition* (December 2014), 17(12): 2769–82.

6 R. Estruch and E. Ros, "Mediterranean Diet for Primary Prevention of Cardiovascular Disease," *New England Journal of Medicine* (August 2013), 369: 672–677; M. Guasch-Ferre, N. Babio, et al., "Dietary Fat Intake and Risk of Cardiovascular Disease and All-Cause Mortality in a Population at High Risk of Cardiovascular Disease," *American Journal of Clinical Nutrition* (December 2015), 102(6): 1563–73.

7 B. Bendinelli, G. Masala, et al., "Fruit, Vegetables, and Olive Oil and Risk of Coronary Heart Disease in Italian Women: The EPI-COR Study," *American Journal of Clinical Nutrition* (February 2011), 93(2): 275–83; G. Buckland, N. Travier, et al., "Olive Oil Intake and Breast Cancer Risk in the Mediterranean Countries of the European Prospective Investigation into Cancer and Nutrition Study," *International Journal of Cancer* (2012), 131: 2465–9.; Y. Bao, J. Han, et al., "Association of Nut Consumption with Total and Cause-Specific Mortality," *New England Journal of Medicine* (November 2013), 369: 2001–2011.

8 Guasch-Ferre, Babio, et al., "Dietary Fat Intake and Risk of Cardiovascular Disease and All-Cause Mortality."

9 Ibid.

10 T.T. Fung, R.M. van Dam, S.E. Hankinson, M. Stampfer, W.C. Willett, and F.B. Hu, "Low-Carbohydrate Diets and All-Cause and Cause-Specific Mortality: Two Cohort Studies," *Annals of Internal Medicine* (September 7, 2010), 153(5): 289–98.

11 S.R. Preis, M.J. Stampfer, et al., "Dietary Protein and Risk of Ischemic Heart Disease in Middle-Aged Men," *American Journal of Clinical Nutrition* (November 2010), 92(5): 1265–1272.

12 P. Lagiou, S. Sandin, et al., "Low Carbohydrate–High Protein Diet

and Incidence of Cardiovascular Disease in Swedish Women: Prospective Cohort Study," *British Medical Journal* 344 (2012).

13 A. Pan, Q. Sun, et al., "Changes in Red Meat Consumption and Subsequent Risk of Type 2 Diabetes Mellitus: Three Cohorts of US Men and Women," *JAMA International Medicine* (2013), 173(14): 1328–35.

14 R.L. Walford, D. Mock, R. Verdery, and T. MacCallum, "Calorie Restriction in Biosphere 2: Alterations in Physiologic, Hematologic, Hormonal, and Biochemical Parameters in Humans Restricted for a 2-Year Period," *Journals of Gerontology* (June 2002), 57(6): B211–24.

15 Ibid.

16 Ibid.; L. Fontana, T.E. Meyer, S. Klein, and J.O. Holloszy, "Long-Term Calorie Restriction Is Highly Effective in Reducing the Risk for Atherosclerosis in Humans," *PNAS* (April 2004), 101(17): 6659–63.

17 D. Ornish, "Intensive Lifestyle Changes for Reversal of Coronary Heart Disease," *JAMA* (December 1998), 280(23): 2001–7.

18 D.M. Ornish, S.E. Brown, L.W. Scherwitz, et al., "Can Lifestyle Changes Reverse Coronary Atherosclerosis? The Lifestyle Heart Trial," *Lancet* (1990), 336: 129–133.

19 K.L. Gould, D. Ornish, L. Scherwitz, et al., "Changes in Myocardial Perfusion Abnormalities by Positron Emission Tomography After Long-Term, Intense Risk Factor Modification," *JAMA* (1995), 274(11): 894–901.

20 L.J. Appel, F.M. Sacks, et al., "Effects of Protein, Monounsaturated Fat, and Carbohydrate Intake on Blood Pressure and Serum Lipids: Results of the OmniHeart Randomized Trial," *JAMA* (November 2005), 294(19): 2455–64; Bendinelli, Masala, et al., "Fruit, Vegetables, and Olive Oil"; G. Buckland et al., "Olive Oil Intake and Mortality Within the Spanish Population (EPIC-Spain)," *American Journal of Clinical Nutrition* (July 2012), 96(1): 142–149; Guasch-Ferre, Babio, et al., "Dietary Fat Intake and Risk of Cardiovascular Disease and All-Cause Mortality."

21 S. Brandhorst, I.Y. Choi, et al., "A Periodic Diet That Mimics Fasting Promotes Multi-System Regeneration, Enhanced Cognitive Performance, and Healthspan," *Cell Metabolism* 22, no 1 (July 2015): 86–99.

22 Ibid.

CHAPTER 10

1 This work is being led by US National Institute on Aging neuroscientist Mark Mattson's lab.

2 C.C. Liu et al., "Apolipoprotein E and Alzheimer Disease: Risk, Mechanisms and Therapy," *Nature Reviews Neurology* 9, no. 2 (February 2013): 106–118.

3 C. Valls-Pedret et al., "Mediterranean Diet and Age-Related Cognitive Decline: A Randomized Clinical Trial," *JAMA Internal Medicine* (July 2015), 175(7): 1094–1103.

4 Ibid.

5 F. Sofi, R. Abbate, G.F. Gensini, A. Casini, "Accruing Evidence on Benefits of Adherence to the Mediterranean Diet on Health: An Updated Systematic Review and Meta-analysis." *American Journal of Clinical Nutrition* 92, no. 5 (November 2010): 1189–1196, DOI: 10.3945/ajcn.2010.29673, Epub September 1, 2010.

6 G.W. Ross et al., "Association of Coffee and Caffeine Intake with the Risk of Parkinson Disease," *JAMA* (May 2000), 283(20): 2674–9.

7 W.M. Fernando et al., "The Role of Dietary Coconut for the Prevention and Treatment of Alzheimer's Disease: Potential Mechanisms of Action," *British Journal of Nutrition* (July 2015), 114(1): 1–14; Y. Hu et al., "Coconut Oil: Non-Alternative Drug Treatment Against Alzheimer Disease," *Nutrición Hospitalaria* (December 2015), 32(6): 2822–7.

8 N.D. Barnard et al., "Saturated and Trans Fats and Dementia: A Systematic Review," *Neurobiology of Aging* (May 2014), 35 Suppl 2: S65–73.

9 M.C. Morris and C.C. Tangney, "Dietary Fat Composition and Dementia Risk," *Neurobiology of Aging* (September 2014), 35 Suppl 2: S59–S64.

10 R. Shah, "The Role of Nutrition and Diet in Alzheimer Disease: A Systematic Review," *Journal of American Medical Directors Association* (June 2013), 14(6): 398–402; S. Lopes da Silva et al., "Plasma Nutrient Status of Patients with Alzheimer's Disease: Systematic Review and Meta-Analysis," *Alzheimer's and Dementia* (July 2014), 10(4): 485–502; M.H. Mohajeri et al., "Inadequate Supply of Vitamins and DHA in the Elderly: Implications for Brain Aging and Alzheimer-Type Dementia," *Nutrition* (February 2015), 31(2): 261–75; E.M. Brouwer-Brolsma and L.C. de Groot, "Vitamin D and Cognition in Older Adults: An Update of Recent Findings," *Current Opinion in Clinical Nutrition and Metabolic Care* (January 2015), 18(1): 11–6; T. Cederholm, N. Salem, Jr., and J. Palmblad, "Çx-3 Fatty Acids in the Prevention of Cognitive Decline in Humans," *Advances in Nutrition* (November 2013), 4(6): 672–6.

11 S. Garcia-Ptacek et al., "Body Mass Index in Dementia," *European Journal of Clinical Nutrition* (November 2014), 68(11): 1204–9.

12 S. Brandhorst et al. and V.D. Longo, "A Periodic Diet That Mimics Fasting Promotes Multi-System Regeneration, Enhanced Cognitive Performance, and Healthspan," *Cell Metabolism* 22, no. 1 (July 2015): 86–99.

13 C. Groot et al., "The Effect of Physical Activity on Cognitive Function in Patients with Dementia: A Meta-Analysis of Randomized Control Trials," *Ageing Research Reviews* (January 2016), 12: 773–783.

14 B.Y. Li et al., "Mental Training for Cognitive Improvement in Elderly People: What Have We Learned from Clinical and Neurophysiologic Studies?" *Current Alzheimer Research* (July 2015), 12(6): 543–52.

CHAPTER 11

1 K.L. Ong et al., "Trends in C-Reactive Protein Levels in US Adults from 1999 to 2010," *American Journal of Epidemiology* (June 2013), 177(12): 1430–42.

2 G.S. Cooper et al., "Recent Insights in the Epidemiology of Auto-immune Diseases: Improved Prevalence Estimates and Under-standing of Clustering of Diseases," *Journal of Autoimmunity* (November–December 2009), 33(3–4): 197–207.

3 A. Lerner, "The World Incidence and Prevalence of Autoimmune Diseases Is Increasing," *International Journal of Celiac Disease* (2015), 3(4): 151–155.

4 A. Manzel et al., "Role of 'Western Diet' in Inflammatory Autoim-mune Diseases," *Current Allergy and Asthma Reports* (January 2014), 14(8): 454.

5 Ibid.

6 A. Lawrence et al., "Diet Rapidly and Reproducibly Alters the Human Gut Microbiome," (January 2014), 505(7484): 559–563.

7 M.M. Lamb et al., "The Effect of Childhood Cow's Milk Intake and HLA-DR Genotype on Risk of Islet Autoimmunity and Type 1 Diabetes: The Diabetes Autoimmunity Study in the Young," *Pedi-atric Diabetes* (February 2015), 16(1): 31–8.

8 S.G. Verza et al., "Immunoadjuvant Activity, Toxicity Assays, and Determination by UPLC/Q-TOF-MS of Triterpenic Saponins from *Chenopodium* Quinoa Seeds," *Journal of Agricultural and Food Chemistry* (March 2012), 60(12): 3113–8.

9 C. Astler et al., "First Case Report of Anaphylaxis to Quinoa, a Novel Food in France," *Allergy* (May 2009), 64(5): 819–20.

10 C-W Cheng et al., "Prolonged Fasting Reduces IGF-1/PKA to Pro-mote Hematopoietic-Stem-Cell-Based Regeneration and Reverse Immunosuppression," *Cell Stem Cell* (June 2014), 14(6): 810–23.

11 I.Y. Choi et al., "A Diet Mimicking Fasting Promotes Regeneration and Reduces Autoimmunity and Multiple Sclerosis Symptoms," *Cell Reports* (June 2016), 15(10): 2136–46.

12 Ibid.

13 H. Müller et al., "Fasting Followed by Vegetarian Diet in Patients with Rheumatoid Arthritis: A Systematic Review," *Scandinavian Journal of Rheumatology* (2001), 30(1): 1–10.

14 J. Kjeldsen-Kragh et al., "Controlled Trial of Fasting and One-Year Vegetarian Diet in Rheumatoid Arthritis," *Lancet* (October 1991), 338(8772): 899–902.

15 Ibid.

16 Müller et al., "Fasting Followed by Vegetarian Diet."

17 Ibid.

Index

Italicized page numbers indicate locations of illustrations, charts, and tables

age, aging, xvii, 4, 6, 12–14, 16–29, 31–34, 53–55, 70, 156, 162–63, 212–13
  acceleration of, 27, 33, 57–58, 66–67, 83–84, 118, 125, 179
  in baker's yeast, 17, 24–28, 31, 66
  calorie restriction and, 24, 57–58
  cancer and, *33, 71,* 79, 118–19, 127, *128, 135*
  causes of, 13–14, 17–21
  CVD and, 165–66, 183
  delaying of, xiv, xviii–xix, 8, 13, 55, *55,* 79, 96
  exercise and, 87–90, 92–94, 190–91
  FMD and, xviii–xix, *99, 100,* 102, *103,* 108, 110–11, *123,* 152, 181–82, 190, 216
  genes and, 10, 17–18, 24–28, 31, 33, 36, 45, 47, 57, 118, 179, 212
  immune system and, 194–95, 206
  link between diet and, 10, 43, 69, 84
  Longevity Diet and, 59–60, 63–64, 71–86, 145, *164,* 214, 220
  Longo's fascination with, xi, xiii
  neurodegenerative diseases and, 176–79, 181–82, 186–88, 190, 192–93
  and Pillars of Longevity, 21–22, 43–45, 47–48, 57, 66–67, 69, *70*
  programmed, 17–18
  programmed longevity and, 19–23, 31
  Prolon and, 98–99
  protecting against, xiv, 17, 19–22, 26–27, 31–32
  risk and, 25, 32, 69, *103, 109,* 152, 170
  slowing it down, 16, 22, 24
  in worms, 26–28
  see also centenarians
alcohol, 29, 55–56, 115, 137, 155
almonds, 5, 60, 70, 76, 83, 146, 165, 174, 214, 233, 242, *259, 263, 265*
  milk and, 4, 223, 225, 231, 234–35, 237, 243, 246, 249, 254, 256, 262, 266
altruistic death program, 18–19
Alzheimer's disease (AD), xvii, 116, 156, 175–93
  diet and, 177–82, 184–89, 191–93
  FMD and, *109,* 177–79, 181–82, 190, 192
  prevention of, 179, 181–84, 186, 189, 191
  risk and, 32, *109,* 116, 178, 182, 185–87, 189–92
  treatment of, 177–81, 185, 188, 192–93
Ames, Bruce, 53
amino acids, 50–51, 112
  aging and, 28, 33, 57, 66
  neurodegenerative diseases and, 179, 189, 192

anchovies, 5, 84, 136, *257, 263*
  pizza with vegetables, anchovies, and
    sardines, 250–51
animal rights activists, 120–21
Army, U.S., 7–9
autoimmune diseases, xii, xvi, 62, 195–210
  diet and, 35, *109*, 111, 197–98, 200–206,
    203, 208–10
  prevention of, 197–200, 210
  risk and, 68, *109*, 197–98
  treatment of, 34–36, 200–210
autophagy, 102, 105–6, 152

bacteria, 12, 61, 195, 197, 203
baker's yeast (*Saccharomyces cerevisiae*),
    96, *256*
  aging in, 17, 24–28, 31, 66
  longevity and, 28–29, *28*
  and Pillars of Longevity, 44–45
Barcelona study, 165, 174–75, 183
barley, 219, 222
  barley salad with broccoli, feta, and
    tomatoes, 249–50
  barley salad with olives and nuts,
    229–30
basic research, *see* juventology/basic
    research
bicycling, 90–91, *93*, 191
Biosphere 2, 24, *25*, 58, 96, 166–67, *167*
blood, blood pressure, 14–15, 68, 80, 97,
    108, 125–26, 155, 195, 202
  cancer and, 132, 135
  CVD and, 160, *167*, 171, *173*
  diabetes and, 139, 148–49, 152, 158
  FMD and, *103*, 104–5, *105*, 109, 112,
    133–34, 152, 157–58, 171–72, *173*, 175
  and food we eat, 50–52
body mass index (BMI), 134, 136, 168,
    187–88, 222*n*, 220
  CVD and, *167*, 174
  diabetes and, 139, *140*, *150*
bones, xiv, 53, 98, *99*, 206
brains, brain, 49, 98, 152
  aging and, 73, 181, 186
  Laron syndrome and, 29–30
  Longevity Diet and, 63, 144
  neurodegenerative diseases and,
    176–78, 181, 183–84, 186–87, 191
breads, 4, 6, 24, 40, 51–52, *114*, 133, 135
  CVD and, 170, 174
  garbanzo bean bread with raw
    vegetables, 228

garbanzo bean salad and vegetables
    with garbanzo bean bread, 238–39
  Longevity Diet and, 60–62, 76, 81–82,
    145, 214–15, 220, 223, 226–29, 232–35,
    238–43, 247–51
  minerals in, *257-59, 266*
  vitamins in, *255*
  whole-grain, 51, 82, 223, 226–27, 233,
    242–43, 247, 249, *258-59, 266*
breakfasts, 6, 85, *114*
  Longevity Diet and, 62–64, 142, 145,
    215, 220, 222–23, 225, 227, 229, 231,
    233, 235, 237, 239, 241, 243, 245,
    247, 249
  minerals in, *256, 258, 266*
  vitamins in, *253-55, 260, 263*
broccoli, 85, *114*, 136, *255, 258-61, 263, 267*
  barley salad with broccoli, feta, and
    tomatoes, 249–50
  broccoli soup, 239
  cream of garbanzo beans + steamed
    broccoli, 248–49
  pasta with broccoli and black
    beans, 224
brussels sprouts, *255, 261*
  brussels sprouts with garlic, pine nuts,
    and Parmesan cheese, 235–36
Buchinger Wilhelmi clinics, 102
Buettner, Dan, 42, 81, 88

Calabria, xii, xv–xvi, 1, 169
  centenarian studies in, 72–73, 88, 211
  diet in, 3–6
calcium, 53, 220, 223, *256-58, 262*
Calment, Jeanne, 75
calories, 6, 40, 43, 46, 56, 93
  autoimmune diseases and, 204, 208–9
  CVD and, 161–62, *167*–68, 174
  diabetes and, 141, 148, 207
  FMD and, 100, 102, *114*, 115, 131, 133, 149,
    151, 158, 181, 204, 209, 216
  Longevity Diet and, 62–63, 71–72, 85,
    143–44, *143*, 215, 220–21, 223, 226, 230,
    232, 234, 236, 238, 240, 242, 244, 246,
    248, 250
  neurodegenerative diseases and,
    181–82, 192
  restriction of, 24, 38, 57–59, 96–97, 141,
    148, 161–63, 167–68, 170, 181–82
Campbell, T. Colin, 67
cancer, xi–xii, xvi–xix, 2, 37, 40, 57, *74*, 80,
    156, 161, 211, 217

aging and, *33, 71,* 79, 118–19, 127, *128, 135*

diet and, xviii–xix, 53, 100, *103, 109,* 111, 113, 120, 122, *123,* 124–34, *128,* 132–37, *135,* 146, 171, 180, 184, 188, 212

fasting and, 36, 97, 122–24, *123,* 126–34, *128, 130,* 207, 212

and guidelines for patients and doctors, 132–33

Laron syndrome people and, 29, *31*

Longevity Diet and, 73, 134–35

in Okinawans vs. Americans, 73, *73*

and Pillars of Longevity, 45, 67–68, 70, *70*

Prolon and, 97–98

protein and, *33,* 38, 67, 70, *70, 71,* 79, 134–35, 146

risk and, 32–33, 67–68, 71, *71,* 73, *73, 103,* 108, *109,* 113, 116, 132, 134, *135,* 136, 171, 184, 195

starving patients with, 119–20, 122–24, *123,* 126–34, *128, 130*

treatment of, xviii–xix, 34–36, 45, *55,* 67, 96–98, 100, 106, 118–37, *123,* 188, 206–7, 212

see also under clinical studies

carbohydrates, 7, 42, 133, 166, 189, 204

complex, 4, 51, 58, 60–61, 67, 71–72, 85, *114,* 143, 145, 214, 220

diet and, 47–48, 60–61, 65–68, *69,* 71–72, 84–85, 143, 145–46, 204, 214–15, 220

exercise and, 94–95

food sources of, 51–52, 60, *114*

and Pillars of Longevity, 47–48, 66–68

cardiovascular disease (CVD), xii–xiii, xvii, 33, 37, 40, *74,* 80, 156, 159–62, 165–75

diet and, 64–65, 70, 73, *103, 109,* 111, 113, 161–62, 165–69, 171–75, *173,* 183, 185–86, 188, 192, 197

and Pillars of Longevity, 46, 68, 170, 173

prevention of, 167, 172–73

risk and, 32, 64–65, 68, 70, *103,* 113, 116, 142, 149, 159, 165–68, *167,* 171–73, *173,* 183–84, 186, 192, 195

treatment of, 36, *55,* 107, 160–61, 168–70, 173–75, 188

carrots, 41, 85, *114,* 136, 226, 228–30, 232–36, 240, 243–45, 247–50, *260, 267*

fennel salad with tomatoes, carrots, onions, and olives, 243

Caruso, Salvatore, 2, 38, 76, *77,* 88, 193, 218

cells, 14, 24, 34, 91, 118–25, 211

aging and, 20, 22, 44, 47

autoimmune diseases and, 196–97, 201–2

cancer and, 96, 118–20, 122–25, 133, 195, 207

diabetes and, 139, 197

fasting and, 99–100, 124

FMD and, 102–3, 105–6, 108–9, 152, 202–4

and food we eat, 50–52

immune system and, 98–99, 194–97, 201–3, *201, 203*

Longevity Diet and, 61, 215

muscles and, 8, 11–12

and Pillars of Longevity, 44, 47

progenitor, 203–4

programmed longevity and, 20–21

regeneration, protection, and repair of, xii, xiv, 20, 22, 36, 44, 152, 156, 171, *201,* 203, *203*

sperm, 19, 104, *104*

see also stem cells

centenarians, 35, 54

CVD and, 73, *74,* 169–70

diets of, 2–6, 64, 71–83, *72,* 163, 169, 217–18

exercise and, 73, 87–88

hot spots for, 42, 81–82

studies on, xi–xii, xv–xvi, 2, 42, *44,* 46, 71–83, *72, 73, 74,* 87–88, 163, 170, 211, 217

cereals, *114*

Longevity Diet and, *164,* 225, 235, 247

minerals in, *256, 258, 266*

vitamins in, *253–55, 260, 263*

cheeses, xiii, 6, 15, 40–41, 56, *114,* 143–45, *143,* 186, 188–89, 192

barley salad with broccoli, feta, and tomatoes, 249–50

brussels sprouts with garlic, pine nuts, and Parmesan cheese, 235–36

Greek salad with feta, olives, onion, and peppers, 237–38

grilled eggplant with feta cheese and tomatoes, 233–34

Longevity Diet and, 59–60, 79, 82, 85, 145, *164,* 214, 224, 228–29, 233–38, 241, 244, 249–50

Chemolieve, xviii–xix, 132

chemotherapy, 34–36, 67, 97, 119–34, 136, *201*, 206–7
    clinical trials on, 129–32, *130*
    side effects of, 126, *128*, 129–32, *130*, 207
    starving cancer patients and, 119–20, 122–24, *123*, 126–34, *128*, *130*
Chicago, xiii, 3, 5–7
chicory, 225, 242–43
China Study, The, 67
chocolate, 188, 217–18, *262*
    Longevity Diet and, 223, 226, 230, 232, 234, 236–38, 240, 242, 244–46, 248, 250
cholesterol, 15, 39, 65, 182
    CVD and, *167*, 169–71, *173*
    FMD and, *103*, 109, *150*, 171–72
    and Pillars of Longevity, 46–47
    treatments for, 107–8
clams, 84, *253*
    spaghetti with clams and mussels, 236–37
clinical studies, xii, xiv–xv, xvii–xix, 4, 40–42, *44*, 45–48, 118, 121, 148, 163, 170, 175, 181, 185, 189–91, 211, 217
    on cancer, xviii, *103*, 118, 120, 125–32, *128*, *130*, 137, 156
    on FMD, xiv, xviii–xix, 42, *103*, 105, 108, 110–12, 127–29, *128*, *130*, 131–32, 134, 137, 149–50, *150*, 152, 158–59, 171–72, 177, 179, 190, 200–202, 204–5, 208–10
    on Longevity Diet, 68–71, 173, 177, 210
coconuts
    milk and, 223, 230, 242, 250, *256*, *262*
    neurodegenerative diseases and, 185–86, 188–89, 191–92
coffee, 4, 42, 56, 115
    Longevity Diet and, 222, 224*n*, 227, 229, 231, 233, 237, 239, 241, 243, 247, 249
    neurodegenerative diseases and, 184–85, 191
colitis, xvii, 62, 208
complex systems, studies of, xv, *44*, 46–47
    exercise and, 89, 91
    Longevity Diet and, 83–84
corn, 5, 52, 162, 229–30, 235, *258*, *263*
corticosteroids, 125
Costa Rica, 72, 88, 163
C-reactive protein (CRP), *103*, *150*, 158, *167*, 171–72, *173*, 195, 209
Crohn's disease, xvii, 62, 195–96, 208–9

Darwin, Charles, 17
deaths, death, 10, 13, 27, 35, 37, 53, 67, 108, 125, 178, 187
    aging and, 17–20, 24
    animal testing and, 120–21
    calorie restriction and, 58, 161–62
    cancer and, *31*, *71*, 146, 207
    CVD and, 160, 165–66
    and dangers of fasting, 153–54
    exercise and, 92–93
    Longevity Diet and, 66, 70
    in Molochio, 1–2, 79
    proteins and, 38, *71*
    risk and, 32, 71, *71*, 93
de Cabo, Rafael, 162
Deiana, Luca, 81
dementias, 73, 175
    diet and, 177, 184–88, 191–92
    exercise and, 190–91
desserts, 5–6, 115
    Longevity Diet and, 224, 226, 229, 231, 233, 235, 237, 239, 241–42, 244, 247, 249, 251
diabetes, xii–xiii, *33*, 40, 57, 80, 137–59, 211
    cautionary tale on, 154–55
    diagnosis of, 138–39, 149
    diet and, 62, 65, *103*, 109, *109*, 111–13, 134, 141–58, *150*, 153, 171, 184, 188, 207
    Laron syndrome people and, 29, *31*, 146–47
    monkeys and, 141, 161–62
    obesity and, 139, 146–48, 157–58
    and Pillars of Longevity, 45–46, 68
    prevention of, 141–48, 151–53, 156, 159, 184
    reversal of, 141, 149–53, *153*
    risk and, 32, 45, 65, 68, *103*, *109*, 113, 116, 138–40, *140*, 146–52, *150*, 157–58, 171, 197
    treatment of, 36, *55*, 109, 142, 147–51, 155–56, 159, 188, 207
    type 1, xvii, 62, 109, 153, *153*, 195–97
    type 2, xvii, 109, 138–40, 149, 153, *153*, 184
diets, dieting, xii–xv, 29, 50–53, 63, 208–12
    aging and, *55*, 66, 163
    in Army, 7–8
    autoimmune diseases and, 35, *109*, 111, 197–98, 200, 202–6, *203*, 208–10
    calorie restriction (CR), 24, 38, 57–59, 96–97, 141, 148, 161–63, 167–68, 170, 181–82

cancer and, xviii–xix, 53, 100, *103*, *109*,
111, 113, 120, 122, *123*, 124–34, *128*,
132–37, *135*, 146, 171, 180, 184, 188, 212
of centenarians, 2–6, 64, 71–83, *72*, 163,
169, 217–18
chemotherapy and, 133, *201*
in Chicago, xiii, 6–7
CVD and, 64–65, 70, 73, *103*, *109*, 111,
113, 161–62, 165–69, 171–75, *173*, 183
185–86, 188, 192, 197
diabetes and, 62, 65, *103*, 109, *109*,
111–13, 134, 141–58, *150*, *153*, 171, 184,
188, 207
and eating at table of your ancestors,
198–200, 210
and eating in moderation, 40–41, 101
exercise and, 87–88, 112–13, 216
genes and, 31–32, 38, 80, 103, 110–12,
134, 153, 181
high-fat, 6, 67–68, 145–46
high-protein, 47–48, 58, 66–68, *69*,
146, 189
high-sugar, 6, 58, 162–63
inflammatory diseases and, 195–97
link between aging, longevity, disease
and, xiii, 4, 10, 37–38, 43, 58, 66–67,
69, 75–76, 83–84, 116, 163
listening to right people on, 39–42, 47
longevity and, xiii, 2–6, 24, 37–44,
47–48, 58, 64, 66–67, 69, *69*, 71–83,
72, 161, 163, 169, 181, 217–18
low-carb, 47–48, 65–68, *69*, 71,
145–46, 204
low-protein, 2, 8, 66–67, 69, *69*, 79,
147, 189
low-sugar, 8, 46
neurodegenerative diseases and, 177–93
obesity and, 113, 133, 152, 157–58
and Pillars of Longevity, 43–48, 57,
66–86, *69*
see also specific diets
differential stress resistance, 36, 45, 119
dinners, 4, 6, 85, *114*, 155
Longevity Diet and, 63–64, 82, 85, 145, 215,
220–21, 223, 226, 228–42, 244, 246–51
disposable soma theory, 19
DNA, 12, 61, 88, 103, 182
aging and, 17, 19–20
autoimmune diseases and, 197–98
cancer and, 118, 124
drugs, 11, 15, 34–36, 80, 106–9, 154, 161,
169, 180

autoimmune diseases and, 206–7
diabetes and, 148–51, 155–56
FMD and, 108–9, 111–12, 134, 158, 175
side effects of, 41, 107
see also chemotherapy

Ecuador, xv, 38, 46, 57
Laron syndrome in, 29–31, *30*, *31*, 77–78,
80, 146–47, 211
eggplant, 246
grilled eggplant with feta cheese and
tomatoes, 233–34
eggs, 6, 39, 41–42, *72*, 75, 167, 188–89,
198, *259*
Longevity Diet and, 59, 72, 79–81, 85,
164, 214
vitamins in, *254*, *256*, *260*, *262*
environment, 12, 18, 24, 62, 84, 124,
166–67, 196
epidemiology, xi–xii, xv, 4, 41, *44*, 45–48,
163, 170, 173, 211–12, 217
exercise and, 91–92
Longevity Diet and, 67–68, 75
escarole, olives, tomatoes, and basil,
231–32
Esselstyn diet, 169–70, 173, 175
evolution, 10–12, 31, 34, 62, 84, 91, 101, 107,
109, 122–24
aging and, 17–18, 20
longevity and, 20, 45
exercise, xv, 7–8, 32, 82, 87–95, *93*, 102
cancer and, 136, 217
centenarians and, 73, 87–88
CVD and, 168, 172, 174
diet and, 87–88, 112–13, 216
neurodegenerative diseases and, 188,
190–91
optimizing of, 89–92

Fabrizio, Paola, 118
fasting, 12, 99–102, 121, 181, 185
autoimmune diseases and, *203*, 206–8
cancer and, 36, 97, 122–24, 126–34, *128*,
130, 207, 212
dangers of, 153–54
diabetes and, 139, 141, 147–49
intermittent, 101–2
Longevity Diet and, 64–65
periodic, prolonged, 100–102
and Pillars of Longevity, 42, 67
side effects of, *128*, 129
water-only, xix, 26, 120, 129, 153–54

fasting-mimicking diets (FMDs), xiv, 32, 35–36, 42, 45, 97–115, *105*, *151*, 154, 163–64, 175–79, 201
  aging and, xviii–xix, *99*, *100*, 102, *103*, 108, 110–11, *123*, 152, 181–82, 190, 216
  autoimmune diseases and, 35, *109*, 111, 200–206, *203*, 208–10
  cancer and, xviii–xix, 100, *103*, *109*, 111, 113, *123*, 124–34, *135*, 136, 171
  CVD and, *103*, *109*, 111, 113, 161, 171–73, *173*, 175
  diabetes and, *103*, 109, *109*, 111–13, 134, 141, 147–53, *150*, *153*, 156–58, 171
  effects on humans of, 102–5, 109
  and guidelines for patients and doctors, 132–34
  Longevity Diet and, 64–65, 86, 102, 114, 171, 204–5, 210, 216
  neurodegenerative diseases and, *109*, 111, 113, 177–79, *180*, 181–83, 190–92
  obesity and, 113, 133, 152, 157–59
  preparation for, 114, *114*
  Prolon and, xix–xx, 97–99, 104, 110, 157, 159
  regenerative self-healing process and, 105–6, 108–9, *109*
  risk and, *103*, 104, 108–9, *109*, 112–13, 115, 133, 182, 190
  side effects of, xix, 114–15, 126, 133, 158, 201, 204–5
  when to start it, 113
  who may do it, 110–11
  who may not do it, 111–12
  see also under clinical studies
fats, fat, 42, 133, 162
  abdominal, xiv, 45, 65, 85–86, 98, 103–4, 115, 139–42, 145, 148, 151, 157–58, 171–72, 187, 196, 210, 215–16, 222*n*
  autoimmune diseases and, 196, 204, 210
  bad, 58, 60, 144–45, 186, 214
  CVD and, 165–66, 169–70, 174–75
  diabetes and, 139–40, 148
  diet and, 6, 8, 47–48, 58, 60, 63, 65, 67–68, *69*, 70–72, 84–86, 97, 103–4, *114*, 115, 142–46, 151–52, 158, 171–72, 186, 210, 214–16, 220–21
  fasting and, 97, 101
  food sources of, 52, *114*
  good, 58, 60, 71, 85, 97, 137, 143–44, 146, 189, 214, 221
  hydrogenated, 60, 214
  monounsaturated, 52, 144, 165, 186

  neurodegenerative diseases and, 185–88, 192
  obesity and, 145, 157–58
  and Pillars of Longevity, 45–47, 68
  polyunsaturated, 52, 165
  saturated, 48, 52, 56, 60, 68, 72, 84–85, *114*, 137, 144, 165, 185–86, 192, 214
  trans, 60, 72, 165, 186, 214
  unsaturated, 52, 60, 214, 221
fennel salad with tomatoes, carrots, onions, and olives, 243
Finch, Caleb, 23, 177
fish and seafood, 4, 52–53, *72*, 162, 188–89, 192, 198
  black/venus rice with zucchini and shrimp, 244
  and cancer, 135–37
  and CVD, 165, 167, 169–70, 174
  and FMD, 114, *114*
  and Longevity Diet, 5, 59–60, 63, 67, 72, 76, 84–85, 114, 214, 221, 226, 232–33, 236–37, 240, 244, 250–51
  minerals in, *256-59, 267*
  octopus with potato, 232–33
  omega-3 in, 84, *264-66*
  pasta with tuna, olives, capers, and tomato, 240
  pizza with vegetables, anchovies, and sardines, 250–51
  salmon fillet with asparagus, 226
  spaghetti with clams and mussels, 236–37
  vitamins in, *253-54, 256, 260, 262-63*
Five Pillars of Longevity, xv, 21–22, 38, 41–48, *55*, *70*, 163–64, 213
  applications of, 43, 47–48, 50
  components of, 44–47, *44*
  and CVD, 46, 68, 170, 173
  and diet, 43–48, 57, 66–86, *69*
  exercise and, 89, 91–92
5:2 diet, 147–49
Fraser, Gary, 82
free radicals, 10, 19, 22, 26
fruit flies, 28–29, *28*, 66
fruits, 5–6, 51, *72*, *114*, 133, 188, 204
  CVD and, 167–69, 174
  juices and, 6, 10, 51, 61, 111, 224*n*, *255*, *257*, 261–62
  Longevity Diet and, 60–61, 72, 81, *164*, 220, 223–24, 226–29, 231, 233, 235, 237, 239, 241–45, 247, 249, 251
  minerals in, *257-59, 267*

spinach with pine nuts and raisins, 223
vitamins in, *255-56, 260-63*

garbanzo beans, 4–5, 40, 85, 136, 143–44,
    174, 198, *256, 259*
    cream of garbanzo beans + steamed
        broccoli, 248–49
    garbanzo bean bread with raw
        vegetables, 228
    garbanzo bean minestrone with pasta,
        228–29
    garbanzo bean salad and vegetables
        with garbanzo bean bread, 238–39
genes, genetics, xiv, 23–34, 41, 62, 87–88,
    146–47, 211–12
    aging and, 10, 17–18, 24–28, 31, 33, 36,
        45, 47, 57, 118, 179, 212
    baker's yeast and, 25–26
    cancer and, 118, 134
    diet and, 31–32, 38, 48, 80, 103, 110–12,
        134, 153, 181
    growth, 28–32, *28, 31*
    longevity and, 23, 27–29, *28,* 31, 33–34, 38
    neurodegenerative diseases and, 178–82
    and Pillars of Longevity, 45, 47–48
Genoa, 13, 39, 90, 120
    diet in, 3–5
    Longo's background in, xii, xv–xvi
Germany, xv, 102, 198, 200
Gilbert, Daniel, 56
glucose, 11, 46, 49, 51, 97, 108, 125–26,
    167, 185
    diabetes and, 139, 141, 147–49, 152,
        154, 158
    FMD and, *103,* 104, 109, 112, 133, 152–53,
        158, 172
glycemic index, 51–52
glycemic load, 51–52
Gracy, Robert, 14–15
grains, *72, 114,* 133, 162, 204
    barley salad with broccoli, feta, and
        tomatoes, 249–50
    barley salad with olives and nuts, 229–30
    black/venus rice with zucchini and
        shrimp, 244
    CVD and, 167–69, 174
    Longevity Diet and, 60, 66, 72, 80, 82,
        85, 145, 214–15, 219–20, 222–23, 225,
        227, 229–32, 234–38, 240–50
    Mediterranean spelt salad with
        artichokes and mushrooms, 245–46
    minerals in, *258-59, 266-67*

rice with zucchini and peas, 241
spelt and zucchini with garlic, olives,
    and parsley, 227
vitamins in, *254-55, 262-63*
whole, 51, 53, 82, 145, 174, 219, 223,
    226–27, 232–34, 236, 238, 240, 242–50,
    258-59, 266
wild rice and green beans with garlic
    and fresh tomato, 225
Gralla, Edith, 24
Greece, 72, *73,* 169
Greek salad with feta, olives, onion, and
    peppers, 237–38
growth hormone (GH), 14–15
    growth hormone receptor (GHR) genes
        and, 31, 57, 146
    growth hormone receptors (GHRs), 29,
        31, 38, 57, 147
Guevara-Aguirre, Jaime, 29, 31

Hall, Stephen, 78
Harvie, Michelle, 148
hazelnuts, 5, 70, 146, 165, 174, 235, 241,
    257, 263
    milks and, 223, 226, 228, 232, 238–40,
        247–48
hyperglycemia, 47, *130*
hypoglycemia, hypoglycemic shock,
    154–56
immune system
    aging and, 194–95, 206
    autoimmune diseases and, 196–97
    cancer and, 124–25, 136, 195
    cells and, 98–99, 194–97, 201–3, *201, 203*
    diet and, 61, 79, 96–97, *100,* 181–82, 197,
        200, 202, *203,* 206
    fasting and, 99, *201, 203,* 206
    neurodegenerative diseases and, 181–82
immunotherapy, 124–25
inflammation, inflammatory diseases,
    98, 171–72
    autoimmune diseases and, 34, 196–97,
        208–9
    immune system and, 194–96
insulin, 51, 57
    and dangers of fasting, 153–54
    diabetes and, 139, 147–48, *153,*
        155–56, 197
    FMD and, 109, 112, 134, 152–53, *153*
    Longevity Diet and, 144, 154
    and Pillars of Longevity, 45, 47
    resistance to, 11, 45, 47, 139, 147, 152

insulin–like growth factor 1 (IGF–1), 57, *203*
  aging and, 66–67, 70, *70*, 79, *135*
  cancer and, 68, *70*, 97, *103*, *135*, 180
  diabetes and, 147, *150*
  FMD and, 97, *103*, 104

Italians, Italy, xi–xiii, xviii, 1–6, 35, 38, 46, 90, 169, 213
  centenarian studies in, xvi, 2, 72–73, *73*, 75–82, 88
  and eating at table of your ancestors, 198–99
  Longo's background in, xii, xv–xvi, 1–4, 6, 13, 75, 198

Japan, xv, 2, 88, 169
  centenarian studies in, 71, *73*, *74*
  and eating at table of your ancestors, 198–99
Johnson, Thomas, 26–27
juices, 204
  fruit, 6, 10, 61, 111, 224*n*
  orange, 10, 51, *255*, *257*, *261-62*
  tomato, *255*, *260-61*
juventology/basic research, xii, xv, xvii–xviii, 21–23, 41, 44–46, *44*, 57, 177, 217
  Longevity Diet and, 66–67

kale, 62, 199–200, 225, *257*
Kenyon, Cynthia, 26
ketogenic diet, 176, 204
ketones, 49, 97, 185
Kirkwood, Tom, 19

lactose intolerance, 62, 198
Laron syndrome, 29–31, *30*, *31*, 77–78, 80, 146–47, 211
Lee, Changhan, 120
legumes, 4–5, 40, 56, 136, 189, 198, 265
  cream of garbanzo beans + steamed broccoli, 248–49
  CVD and, 166–69, 174
  garbanzo bean bread with raw vegetables, 228
  garbanzo bean minestrone with pasta, 228–29
  garbanzo bean salad and vegetables with garbanzo bean bread, 238–39
  Longevity Diet and, 5, 60–61, 63, 72, 76–77, 81–83, 85, 143–45, *164*, 224–25,

228–31, 234–35, 238–39, 241–42, 246, 248–49
  minerals in, *256-59*, *266-67*
  pasta and lentil soup, 230–31
  pasta e vaianeia, 4, 76, 234–35
  pasta with broccoli and black beans, 224
  rice with zucchini and peas, 241
  vitamins in, *255*, *260-61*
  white bean salad with onion, rosemary, and chicory, 242
  wild rice and green beans with garlic and fresh tomato, 225
lifespan, *see* longevity
liver, 98, 145, 184, 195, 205
  diabetes and, 139, 155
  FMD and, 111, 133, 151–52
L-Nutra, xviii–xx, 110, 156
Loma Linda, Calif., 71–73, 82–83, 88, 163, 169
longevity, xi–xv, 33–49, 98, 184, 199
  aging and, 17–23, 28–29, 31
  diet and, xiii, 2–6, 24, 37–44, 47–48, 58, 64, 66–67, 69, *69*, 71–83, *72*, 161, 163, 169, 181, 217–18
  exercise and, 73, 87–92, 216
  extension of, 10, 18, 21–22, 36–38, 41, *55*, 67
  genes and, 23, 27–29, *28*, 31, 33–34, 38
  healthy, xii, xiv–xv, 18, 22–23, 35–39, 41, 44, 47, 49, 54, 56, 59, 63, 65, 73, 146, 211–13, 217
  programmed, 19–23, 31, 33, 35
  social aspects of, 217–18
  solving medical problems and, 34–35
  see also centenarians
Longevity Diet, 5, 52–53, 59–86, *69*, 108, 115, 161–65, 177, 199
  autoimmune diseases and, 204–5, 209–10
  cancer and, 73, *74*, 134–35
  cautionary tale on, 154–55
  comparisons between Mediterranean and, 163–65, *164*
  CVD and, 161, 165, 172–73
  diabetes and, 62, 65, 141–47, 154–56
  eating foods from your ancestry in, 61–62, 85, 215
  eating more, not less, but better in, 143–47, *143*
  eating twice a day plus snack in, 62–64, 85, 144–45, 215

FMD and, 64–65, 86, 102, 114, 171,
  204–5, 210, 216
negative reactions to, 55–56
neurodegenerative diseases and,
  183–84, 186, 188–89, 191, 193
nourishment in, 61, 63, 68
recipes for, 222–51
summaries on, 84–86, 214–16
time-restricted eating in, 64, 70–72, 83,
  86, 142, 164, 215–16, 221
two-week meal plan for, 219–51
lunches, 4, 6, 85, 114, 155
  Longevity Diet and, 63–64, 145,
    220–21, 223, 225, 227, 229–41, 243,
    245–50

mackerel, 59, 253, 264
magnesium, 53, 220, 266–67
meats, xiii, 4, 6–8, 15, 50, 72, 189, 198
  CVD and, 166–67, 169, 174
  diabetes and, 154–55
  Longevity Diet and, 60, 72, 77, 79–80,
    85, 164
  red, 42–43, 56, 60, 166, 174, 186
  white, 60, 85
Mediterranean diet, 101
  autoimmune diseases and, 204, 209
  comparisons between Longevity and,
    163–65, 164
  CVD and, 70, 165, 183
  inflammatory diseases and, 195–96
Mediterranean spelt salad with
  artichokes and mushrooms,
    245–46
medium-chain fatty acids (MCFA),
  185–86
metabolic equivalent tasks (METs),
  92–93, 93
metabolic syndrome, 149, 150
metformin, 112, 134, 155
mice, 10, 30, 35, 48, 106, 211
  aging in, 24–26, 28, 57–58, 66
  autoimmune diseases and, 200–203,
    206, 208
  calorie restriction and, 24, 58, 96–97
  cancer and, 33, 120–21, 123, 125–27,
    136, 180
  diabetes and, 147, 149, 153, 153
  fasting and, 97, 99–100, 206
  FMD and, 99, 100, 100, 105, 109, 123,
    151–53, 153, 180, 190, 202–5
  longevity diets for, 37–38, 66, 69

longevity in, 21, 28–29, 28
neurodegenerative diseases and,
  178–81, 183, 188–90
and Pillars of Longevity, 44–45,
  66–67, 69
Prolon and, 98–99
micronutrients, 52–53, 219
Milan, xi–xii, xviii, 39, 212
mild cognitive impairment, 188
milks, 4–6, 41, 114, 162, 186
  almond, 4, 223, 225, 231, 234–35, 237,
    243, 246, 249, 254, 256, 262, 266
  autoimmune diseases and, 197–98
  coconut, 223, 230, 242, 250, 256, 262
  diabetes and, 154–55
  and eating at table of your ancestors,
    198–99
  of goats, 4–5, 59, 82, 167, 192, 199, 214,
    236, 244
  hazelnut, 223, 226, 228, 232, 238–40,
    247–48
  Longevity Diet and, 59, 62, 79, 82,
    164, 214, 223, 226, 228, 230, 232, 234,
    236–40, 242, 244, 246–50
  neurodegenerative diseases and,
    189, 192
  soy, 256, 262, 266
minerals, 133, 136, 162, 192
  FMD and, 100, 114
  food sources of, 53–54, 256–59,
    266–67
  Longevity Diet and, 61, 85, 143–44, 215,
    219–20, 224, 231, 237, 244, 251
minestrone, 4, 80
  garbanzo bean minestrone with pasta,
    228–29
  Ligurian minestrone, 246–47
Mirisola, Mario, 118
moderation, eating in, 40–41, 101, 188
Molochio, 1–5, 75–79, 234
  centenarian studies in, 2, 76, 78, 81
  fountain plaza of, 1–2, 3
monkeys, 21, 141
  diets and, 37–38, 58, 96–97, 161–63, 167
  exercise and, 87–88
Morano, Emma, 38, 78, 79–81, 193
Mosley, Michael, 148
multiple sclerosis (MS), xvii, 195–96, 211
  symptoms of, 202–3, 208
  treatment of, 34, 200–205, 208–9
multivitamins, 53, 61, 85, 114, 114, 192, 215,
  220, 224, 231, 237, 244, 251

muscles, xiv, 11–12, 98, 139, 141, 146
  exercise and, 8, 91–95, 216
  FMD and, *103*, 152, 182
  and food we eat, 50–51, 59–60
  Longevity Diet and, 59–60, 62–63, 71,
    79, 85, 214–15, 220–21
  neurodegenerative diseases and, 182,
    188–89
mushrooms, *114*, 229–30, 236, 250, 262-63
  Mediterranean spelt salad with
    artichokes and mushrooms, 245–46
music
  comparisons between science and, 9–11
  Longo's education and career in, xi,
    xiii, 5–7, 9–12, 23
mussels, 5, *253*, *258*, *264*
  spaghetti with clams and mussels,
    236–37
mutations, 80, 87, 134
  cancer and, 118, 124
  FMD and, 110–12
  growth genes and, 28–31, *28*, *30*, *31*
  Laron syndrome and, 30, *30*, *31*, 146, 211
  neurodegenerative diseases and, 178–79

neurodegenerative diseases, xii, xvi, 36,
    175–93
  diet and, 177–93
  exercise and, 188, 190–91
  FMD and, *109*, 111, 113, 177–79, *180*,
    181–83, 190–92
  risk and, 32, *109*, 113, 116, 178, 182–87,
    189–92
nutraceuticals, 180–81
nutritechnologies, 8, 50, 97, 180–81
nuts, 4–5, 53, 56, *114*, 137, *265*
  barley salad with olives and nuts, 229–30
  brussels sprouts with garlic, pine nuts,
    and Parmesan cheese, 235–36
  CVD and, 165–67, 169–70, 174–75, 183
  Longevity Diet and, 60, 67, 70, 72, 76,
    82–83, 85, 146, 165, 214, 223, 225–44,
    246–51
  minerals in, *256-59*, *266*
  neurodegenerative diseases and,
    183–84, 191
  spinach with pine nuts and raisins, 223
  vitamins in, *254-55*, *260*, *262-63*

oats, oatmeal, 231, 237, *266-67*
obesity, 6, *31*, 32, 41, 80, 145, 156–59,
    195–96

case studies on, 157–59
diabetes and, 139, 146–48, 157–58
diet and, 63, 113, 133, 152, 157–59
octopus, *264*
  octopus with potato, 232–33
oils, 232, *263*
  coconut, 185–86, 188–89, 191–92
  CVD and, 165, 169
  omega-3 in, *265-66*
Okinawans, Okinawa, xv, 169
  cancer and, 73, *73*, 74
  centenarian studies in, 2, 42, 71–74, *72*,
    73, *74*, 88, 211
  diet in, 71–73, *72*, 163
  exercise and, *73*, 88
  spirituality of, 74–75
olive oil, 4–5, 52, 56, *114*, 137, *143*, 198
  CVD and, 165, 169–70, 174–75, 183
  Longevity Diet and, 5, 60, 67, 70, 76, 85,
    143–44, 146, *164*, 165, 223–51
  neurodegenerative diseases and,
    183–84, 186, 188, 191
olives, 4
  barley salad with olives and nuts,
    229–30
  escarole, olives, tomatoes, and basil,
    231–32
  fennel salad with tomatoes, carrots,
    onions, and olives, 243
  Greek salad with feta, olives, onion,
    and peppers, 237–38
  Longevity Diet and, 76, 227, 229–33,
    237–38, 240, 243, 245, 251
  pasta with tuna, olives, capers, and
    tomato, 240
  spelt and zucchini with garlic, olives,
    and parsley, 227
omega-3 fatty acid, 52, 61, 82, 114, *114*,
    136, 170, 204, 215, 220, 223, 231, 237,
    244, 251
  food sources of, *72*, 84, *264-66*
  neurodegenerative diseases and, 186,
    189, 192
omega-6 fatty acid, 52, 61, 84, *114*, 136, 215
oocytes, 19, 104, *104*
oranges, 174
  juice and, 10, 51, *255*, *257*, *261-62*
Ornish diet, 168–70, 173–75
overweight, 6, 80, 136
  diabetes and, 139, 147–48
  FMD and, 113, 152, 172–73
  Longevity Diet and, 63, 85

oxygen, oxidation, 19, 22, 27, 61
oysters, *253, 258, 264*

pancreas, 51–52, 99, 131
   diabetes and, 109, 139, 149, *153*, 197
   FMD and, 152–53, *153*
Panda, Satchidananda, 70–71
Parkinson's disease, xvii, 176–77, 184
Passarino, Giuseppe, 78
pasta, 6, 39, 41, 56, *114*, 133, 135, *143*
   CVD and, 170, 174
   garbanzo bean minestrone with pasta,
      228–29
   Longevity Diet and, 60–62, 66, 76, 143,
      145, 214, 219–20, 224, 228–31, 234–37,
      240, 246–47
   pasta and lentil soup, 230–31
   pasta e vaianeia, 4, 76, 234–35
   pasta with broccoli and black
      beans, 224
   pasta with tuna, olives, capers, and
      tomato, 240
   spaghetti with clams and mussels,
      236–37
peanuts, 5, 167, 255, 257–59, 263, 266
peas, 136, 167, 174, 224*n*, 246, *260, 265*
   green, 85, *255, 259, 261*
   rice with zucchini and peas, 241
pecans, 229–30, 239, *265*
peppers, *143*, 224, 229–30, 235–38, 250
   Greek salad with feta, olives, onion,
      and peppers, 237–38
   green, 4, 136, 226, 229, 238, *261*
   red, 236, 238, *260, 261*
Pes, Gianni, 42, 81
pescetarian diets, 3, 59
physical activity levels (PALs), 42, 221
pistachios, 251, *257, 259, 260*
pizza, 6, 143
   pizza with vegetables, anchovies, and
      sardines, 250–51
potatoes, 66, 72, 167, 204, 230, 232–34,
      246–48, *259, 261, 266*
   octopus with potato, 232–33
Poulain, Michel, 42, 81
pregnancy, 49, 111
ProLon, Prolon, xviii–xx, 159
   FMD and, xix–xx, 97–99, 104, 110,
      157, 159
proteins, protein, 40, 133, 162–63, 200, 204
   age and, 14, 28, 33, *33*, 44, 48, 57–58,
      66–67, 70, *70, 71*

cancer and, *33*, 38, 67, 70, *70, 71*, 79,
      134–35, 146
   CVD and, 68, 166, 170, 174
   damaging of, 14–15
   diabetes and, *33*, 68, 146–48
   diet and, 2, 7–8, 47–48, 57–60, 66–69,
      69, 71–72, 79, 83–85, 114, 135, 143–44,
      146–47, *164*, 189, 214–15, 220–21
   exercise and, 91, 94–95, 216
   FMD and, 97, 103, 105, 114, *114*
   food sources of, 50–51, 60, 114, *114*
   as good and bad, 42–43
   neurodegenerative diseases and,
      177–78, 180, 188–90, 192
   and Pillars of Longevity, 44, 47–48,
      66–69
pumpkins, *114, 260, 265*
   pumpkin soup with croutons, 239–40

Quinn, Nora, 126
quinoa, 62, 199–200

Raffaghello, Lizzia, 35, 120
reproduction, 19–20
rheumatoid arthritis (RA), 196, 200,
   208–9
rice, *114*, 133, 204
   black/venus rice with zucchini and
      shrimp, 244
   Longevity Diet and, 60–61, 66, 80, 145,
      214–15, 219, 225, 244
   minerals in, *259, 266-67*
   rice with zucchini and peas, 241
   vitamins in, *254-55, 262*
   wild rice and green beans with garlic
      and fresh tomato, 225
risk, risk factors, xiv, 18, 43, 125
   aging and, 25, 32, 69, *103, 109*, 152, 170
   autoimmune diseases and, 68, *109*,
      197–98
   calorie restriction and, 58, 96–97
   cancer and, 32–33, 67–68, 71, *71*, 73, *73*,
      103, 108, *109*, 113, 116, 132, 134, *135*, 136,
      171, 184, 195
   CVD and, 32, 64–65, 68, 70, *103*, 113,
      116, 142, 149, 159, 165–68, *167*, 171–73,
      173, 183–84, 186, 192, 195
   death and, 32, 71, *71*, 93
   diabetes and, 32, 45, 65, 68, *103, 109*, 113,
      116, 138–40, *140*, 146–52, *150*, 157–58,
      171, 197
   exercise and, 32, 89–90, 93

risk, risk factors (*cont.*)
  FMD and, *103*, 104, 108–9, 112–13, 115,
    133, 182, 190
  Longevity Diet and, 64–65, 67, 70, 108
  neurodegenerative diseases and, 32,
    109, 113, 116, 178, 182–87, 189–92
  and Pillars of Longevity, 45–46, 68–70
  running, 7, 89–91, *93*, 102, 155, 190–91
  Russell, Jenni, 205–7
  Ruvkun, Gary, 28

salads, 41, 146, 226, 229–33, 235–40,
    242–50
  barley salad with broccoli, feta, and
    tomatoes, 249–50
  barley salad with olives and nuts,
    229–30
  escarole, olives, tomatoes, and basil,
    231–32
  fennel salad with tomatoes, carrots,
    onions, and olives, 243
  garbanzo bean salad and vegetables
    with garbanzo bean bread, 238–39
  Greek salad with feta, olives, onion,
    and peppers, 237–38
  Mediterranean spelt salad with
    artichokes and mushrooms, 245–46
  white bean salad with onion, rosemary,
    and chicory, 242
Salazar Aguilar, Freddi, *30*
salmon, 52, 60, 84, 136, 170, 189, 214, *254*,
    257, *260*, *262*, *264*, *266–67*
  salmon fillet with asparagus, 226
  salt, 4, *258*, *264*
  autoimmune diseases and, 197, 210
  Longevity Diet and, 223–30, 232–51
Sanchez Romero, Luis, *30*
sardines, 84, *253*, *256*, *259*, *262*, *264*, *266*
  pizza with vegetables, anchovies, and
    sardines, 250–51
Sardinia, 72–73, 81–82, 88, 169
seafood, *see* fish and seafood
seaweeds, *72*, 198, *258*
sensitization, 36, 45, 155
Seventh-day Adventists, 82, 88, 169
sex, 55–56, 76
shrimp, 84, *264*
  black/venus rice with zucchini and
    shrimp, 244
sleep, 49, 64, 70, 142, 148, 206
smoking, 29, 75–76
smoothies, 5, 228, 240

snacks, xiii, 5, *114*, 174
  Longevity Diet and, 62–64, 85, 142,
    144–45, 215, 220, 223, 226, 228, 230,
    232, 234, 236, 238, 240, 242, 244, 246,
    248, 250
soft drinks, 6–7, 41, 51, 145
soups, 4, 80–81
  broccoli soup, 239
  garbanzo bean minestrone with pasta,
    228–29
  Ligurian minestrone, 246–47
  pasta and lentil soup, 230–31
  pumpkin soup with croutons,
    239–40
  tomato soup with basil, pesto, and
    croutons, 247–48
soy products, *72*, 162, 168, *254*, *265*
  milk and, *256*, *262*, *266*
  vitamins in, *262–63*
spaghetti, *255*, *259*
  spaghetti with clams and mussels,
    236–37
spelt, 223
  Mediterranean spelt salad with
    artichokes and mushrooms, 245–46
  spelt and zucchini with garlic, olives,
    and parsley, 227
spinach, 238–39, *250*, *255*, *259–61*, *263*, *266*
  spinach with pine nuts and raisins, 223
spirituality, 74–75, 217
statins, 15, 107, 109
steaks, 4, 41, 50
stem cells, xiv, 98
  autoimmune diseases and, 202–3, *203*
  fasting and, 99–100, 206
  FMD and, 103, 105–6, *105*, 115, 152,
    202, *203*
  therapies based on, 106–8
sugars, xiii, 5–8, 56, 158
  aging and, 27–28, 33, *33*, 44, 57–58, 67
  cancer and, 134–35
  CVD and, 168, 174
  diet and, 7–8, 46, 51–52, 57–58, 60–62,
    72, 84–86, 96–97, 112, 115, 144–45, 155,
    162–63, 214–15, 220, 223, 224*n*,
    226–27, 229–30, 232, 234, 236, 238–40,
    242, 244, 246, 248, 250
  and Pillars of Longevity, 44–47, 67
supplements, 10, 53–54, 136, *265–66*
  FMD and, 114, *114*, 204
  Longevity Diet and, 61, 85, 114, 215, 220,
    223–24, 231, 237, 244, 251

neurodegenerative diseases and,
186–87, 192
sweet potatoes, 198, *258, 260*
swimming, 91, 191

tea, 4, *114,* 204, 207
  Longevity Diet and, 224*n,* 225, 227, 229,
232, 237, 239, 241, 245, 247, 249
Tex–Mex, 15
tomatoes, 4, 76, 85, *114,* 136, *143,* 198, 225–
27, 229–36, *253, 259, 263*
  barley salad with broccoli, feta, and
tomatoes, 249–50
  cherry, 227, 232–33, 238, 242–45,
249–50
  escarole, olives, tomatoes, and basil,
231–32
  fennel salad with tomatoes, carrots,
onions, and olives, 243
  grilled eggplant with feta cheese and
tomatoes, 233–34
  juice and, *255, 260-61*
  pasta with tuna, olives, capers, and
tomato, 240
  tomato soup with basil, pesto, and
croutons, 247–48
  wild rice and green beans with garlic
and fresh tomato, 225
triglycerides, 52, *167*
  FMD and, *103, 150,* 171–72
Trochon, Jean-Jacques, 126–27
trout, 84, *254, 257, 262, 265*
tuna, 59, *253-54, 259-60, 262, 265*
  pasta with tuna, olives, capers, and
tomato, 240

Valentine, Joan, 24
vegans, veganism, 53, 84, 214
vegetables, 4–5, 51, 53, 56, 133
  barley salad with broccoli, feta, and
tomatoes, 249–50
  barley salad with olives and nuts,
229–30
  black/venus rice with zucchini and
shrimp, 244
  broccoli soup, 239
  brussels sprouts with garlic, pine nuts,
and Parmesan cheese, 235–36
  cancer and, 136–37
  cream of garbanzo beans + steamed
broccoli, 248–49
  CVD and, 165–69, 174

  escarole, olives, tomatoes, and basil,
231–32
  fennel salad with tomatoes, carrots,
onions, and olives, 243
  FMD and, 114, *114,* 204
  garbanzo bean bread with raw
vegetables, 228
  garbanzo bean salad and vegetables
with garbanzo bean bread, 238–39
  Greek salad with feta, olives, onion,
and peppers, 237–38
  grilled eggplant with feta cheese and
tomatoes, 233–34
  Longevity Diet and, 5, 59–61, 63, 67, 72,
72, 76, 79, 82–85, 114, 143–45, 214–15,
220, 223–51
  Mediterranean spelt salad with
artichokes and mushrooms, 245–46
  minerals in, *256-59, 266*
  octopus with potato, 232–33
  pasta with broccoli and black
beans, 224
  pasta with tuna, olives, capers, and
tomato, 240
  pizza with vegetables, anchovies, and
sardines, 250–51
  pumpkin soup with croutons, 239–40
  rice with zucchini and peas, 241
  salmon fillet with asparagus, 226
  spelt and zucchini with garlic, olives,
and parsley, 227
  spinach with pine nuts and raisins, 223
  tomato soup with basil, pesto, and
croutons, 247–48
  vitamins in, *255, 260-61, 263*
  white bean salad with onion, rosemary,
and chicory, 242
  wild rice and green beans with garlic
and fresh tomato, 225
vegetarianism, 82, *167,* 208, *254, 260*
viruses, 61, 195, 203
vitamins, 162, 200
  A, 53, 187, 220, *260, 262*
  B, 53, 84, 186–87, 192, 198, 220, 223, *253-
56, 262*
  C, 10, 22, 136, 181, 186–87, 192, 220, *261*
  D, 53, 68, 186, 192, 220, 223, *256, 262*
  E (alpha–tocopherol), 53, 186–87, 192,
220, *256, 263-64*
  FMD and, 100, 114, *114, 133*
  food sources of, *53-54,* 84, *253-56,
260-63*

vitamins (*cont.*)
    Longevity Diet and, 61, 84–85,
        143–44, 215, 219–20, 223–24, 231, 237,
        244, 251
    neurodegenerative diseases and,
        186–87, 192

Walford, Roy, xiii–xiv, 15, 23–24, *25*, 34,
    44–45, 58, 96, 166–67, 173
walking, 88–91, *93*, 94, 102, 112, 154–55,
    177, 216–17
Wallace, Alfred, 17
walnuts, 4–5, 60, 70, 76, 83, 146, 165, 174,
    214, 224, 231, 237, 239, 243–44, *265*
weight, 40, 97, 162, 174
    cancer and, 135–36
    diabetes and, 141–42
    FMD and, *103*, 110–11, 113, 171, 173,
        182, 190
    Longevity Diet and, 62–63, 65, 71, 79,
        82, 84–86, 135, 142, 145, 210, 214–16,
        220–21, 222*n*
    neurodegenerative diseases and, 182,
        187, 189–90
    see also obesity; overweight
weight gain, 43, 49, 158–59, 163

diabetes and, 154–55
    Longevity Diet and, 220–21, 222*n*
weight loss, 41, 90, 98, 146, 148,
    168, 190, 207
    cancer and, 120, 134, 212, 217
    FMD and, *103*, 133, 151, *151*, 157–59
    Longevity Diet and, 59, 63–64, 142,
        144–45, 214, 222*n*
    obesity and, 157–58
    and Pillars of Longevity, 47–48
weight training, 94–95, 216
Weindruch, Richard, 161
Wilcox, Craig, 42, 72–74
wine, 4, 57, 75–76, *164*, 236
Wisconsin, University of, 161–63
worms, 26–28

yogurts, 157, 167, 188, 236, 244, *260*
    Longevity Diet and, 59, *164*, 214

zucchini, 39, 234, 246
    black/venus rice with zucchini and
        shrimp, 244
    rice with zucchini and peas, 241
    spelt and zucchini with garlic, olives,
        and parsley, 227